TWELVE POWERS OF THE FEMININE AND HOW TO CHANGE THE WORLD

CATHERINE STONE

Twelve Powers of the Feminine
and How to Change the World

First edition, November 2024

ISBN: 9798863271040

TWELVE POWERS OF THE FEMININE AND HOW TO CHANGE THE WORLD

Table *of* Contents

Preface

I present here my experience and understanding of polarity gathered from over 30 years of exploring and observing people and life, and in working with the psyche and the body in my therapy practice with clients.

My training in Polarity Therapy many years ago was a real awakening for me. In later life, marriage and motherhood took me on another incredible journey, but it was my discovery of Tantra, in 2017, that reignited my passion about the wonders of the five elements and polarity. This three-year journey enabled me to go deeper into my understanding of polarity and the feminine and masculine principles.

A few weeks before the Tantra course began, I came to realise that the feminine had become stuck. Or had it? We seemed to be stuck back with the Suffragette movement – still fighting about women's rights while the feminine force within women and men is still unappreciated, denied or suppressed. I found it confusing. I then realised that the former was like a smokescreen over the latter – a "presentation" of the rise of the feminine with the real feminine still repressed behind that mask. But no one seemed to have noticed this.

I felt like I had discovered a terrible secret. One that we are all party to; but that if I uttered my thoughts I'd probably be burnt at the stake – but by women this time. I could see that something was wrong with how we, generally in the West, were still not really *seeing* the feminine. We were *still* not valuing it at all.

Imagine my surprise when here I am but two weeks later after my own realisation about the state of the feminine, seated in front of my new Tantric teacher – a man – and he says, "The feminine revolution has not yet begun... the Suffragette movement wasn't it."

The whole room stopped breathing. The discomfort was tangible. I could feel my eyes were wide. People began to shift uncomfortably on their yoga mats. But I felt electrified and thought I might pop with excitement. This book had begun.

Within a few weeks or so, having begun writing again, I was on the phone to that very Tantra school, and when I said my name as part of my enquiry, she said, "Ooo! Are you an author?" I was stunned. I explained that I actually wasn't *officially*, but that I had felt strongly drawn to write and had just started writing a new manuscript about polarity. She was as surprised as I was and she had no idea why she had asked such a thing. We acknowledged the synchronicity of that moment. That was four years ago and this is three manuscripts and numerous edits later.

For two years at my Tantra class I sat each week submerged in the very material I had learned nearly 30 years previously. Whereas I thought I was just going to be learning some techniques to deepen my connection with my yoni, maybe with some breathing exercises and yoga - while this was true - I also found myself reintroduced to my dear old friends; the five elements of ether, air, fire, water and earth. These fundamental energies of creation weave energy into form, and between them form the neutral, masculine and feminine principles. I already was an expert on the five elements, bolstered by spending 10 years going through the whole body and logging how each organ and system and our whole psyche is underpinned by these energies. (I talk about them throughout the book – especially Earth, Water and Fire as these specifically pertain to the feminine and masculine principles.)

So here I was being given a two-year review by a teacher who clearly knew as much as I did about these elements and how they manifest in the body and psyche. I couldn't believe the synchronicity of this occurrence. Something seemed to be pushing me forward to publish something about this!

The title of this book came to me right at the very end of a different book entirely. I had literally got to the bottom of the last page and put the full stop in and there it appeared: "The Powers of the Feminine and How to Change the World". After writing the first draft I then hesitated for several weeks while dear friends read the manuscript. There was so much more to add; it was as if writing that manifestation of the book primed me for writing this one.

In this book I focus particularly on the feminine principle as this is the force that is naturally more hidden and so most misunderstood (in my experience). Herein I write about the many powers or "ways" of the feminine that together form a very different kind of power to the "empowered woman" we are sold.

When I asked a Facebook group, "What does femininity mean to you?" someone replied, "To be pretty, delicate, weak, small, effete, dependent. Power can be feminine but only through seduction and manipulation, as opposed to masculine power of strength and reason." Well, there it is. Yes, we are very much shown this and taught this. Few women seem to know of the real magic that lies in their femininity. The masculine qualities are therefore shown to be the winner here and are more actively encouraged and aspired to (even though equally misunderstood).

So we are taught masculine = strong and reasonable, feminine = weak and manipulative. Which would you aspire to become?

I teach women about the *real* feminine powers. I show how feminine powers are many, various and incredible! I show that by their very nature they are less obvious than male powers. They are so normal and "everyday" and naturally part of our being that we don't even notice we have them!

But men notice our power. Not necessarily consciously, but

men are affected by the powers of the feminine on a daily basis in both good and bad ways. I have seen how the real feminine powers, in both men and women, are very different from masculine power – also in both men and women. It is the feminine powers that make the world a better place and it is the feminine powers that put women in a place of influence that is transforming, and will continue to truly transform, the world and bring about a New Earth.

"Twelve Powers of the Feminine" is a book to show how women in particular (but not exclusively) can use their feminine incarnation to bring about a future that is good for all of us.

Introduction

Polarity and the Principles

The universe is made of polarity! Everything in the universe has its polar opposite right there alongside it. Light and dark, hot and cold, in and out... Without the polar opposites we have just one big homogeneous sea of nothing. Polarity is what helps create the multitude of "things" that we see and experience within the universe.

Magnetic	Expansive
down	up
in	out
cold	hot
dark	light
returning	going out
listening	speaking
catching	throwing
Shakti	Shiva
egg	sperm
Yin	Yang

The two opposing forces are present in everything. One of the forces is *magnetic* in nature and the other *expansive*. In ancient Chinese tradition, these two opposing qualities have been called Yin and Yang. The Tantrics call them Shakti and Shiva; Shakti being the Goddess – the many forms that consciousness takes - with Shiva being the expansiveness and God-like Pure Consciousness. They have also been known as the feminine and masculine principles.

19

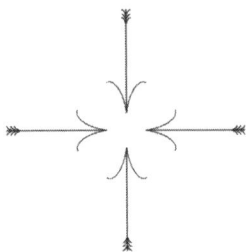 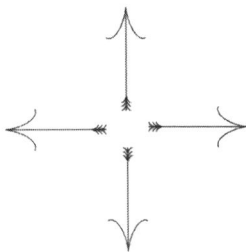

Contracting   Expanding

Neither of these forces is better than the other. Neither force is more powerful than the other. They can both be problematic and they can both be amazing. Both forces have their tendencies and create specific results.

The masculine and feminine principles form the whole of creation. This book shines a light particularly on the feminine principle, but because the feminine does not exist without the masculine, I will also show you how you can recognise the masculine within you. For it is the masculine energy that protects you as a woman and actually *enables* you to unfold fully into your feminine.

The Five Elements

Understanding the five elements and the nature of these different energies is part of understanding the principles and gaining insight into our self as a woman - and indeed the masculine, whether it's the inner masculine or the men in our life. Here is a very simple introduction to these special energies that exist within the whole of creation:

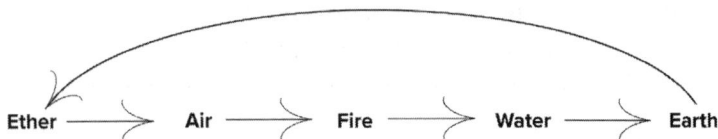

Ether
The space. The space that everything is in. All spaces in the body and mind, space for our feelings, space to think, the throat; grief and expression. Forms the neutral principle with air.

↓

Air
The movement. Denser than ether. All gases. All gases in the body and airiness in the mind, all movement, regulation and balance, the breath, heart-felt feelings, love. Forms the neutral principle with ether.

↓

Fire
The Direction. Denser than air. All direction and all heat and action in the body and mind, all digestion and metabolism, fiery emotions, empowerment, determination and motivation. Masculine principle.

↓

Water
The grounding. Denser than fire. All fluid and fluidity in the body, mind and psyche. All emotional expression, receptivity and flow. Nurturing and creativity. Forms the feminine principle with earth.

↓

Earth
The ground itself. The most dense of all the elements. All structures in the body and mind. All form and completion. The bones. Containment. Survival and safety and emotion of fear. Forms the feminine principle with water.

Ether ⎫
      ⎬ Connected to the neutral principle of balance and purity
Air   ⎭

Fire ⟩ Connected to the masculine principle of direction and action

Water ⎫
       ⎬ Connected to the feminine principle of flow, grounding,
Earth ⎭   structure and form

The Feminine and Masculine Principles

In Tantric teachings it is said that all human beings get to incarnate as a representative of one of the principles, and that hidden within is a spark of the other. If we incarnate as a manifestation of the feminine principle, hidden within is the spark of the masculine. And conversely, if a soul incarnates as the masculine principle - within there is a spark of the feminine. We see this clearly shown in the Taoist symbol of Yin and Yang.

Yin and Yang

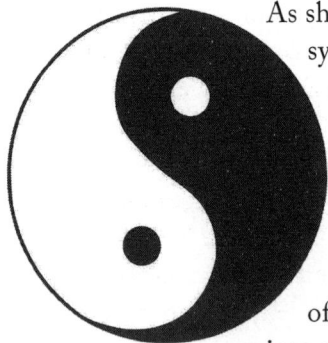

As shown in the Yin and Yang symbol, each principle holds a spark of the other principle within it.

So some of us get to incarnate as a representative of Shakti and some of us get to incarnate as a representative of Shiva. How much we embody into our Shakti or Shiva and how much we embody into our polar opposite is the thing. In health, it's quite a fine balance and this is the journey...

22

Shiva and Shakti

The universal law of polarity is on a different level to that of identity. Anything to do with our identity is more to do with the ego level and our sense of self. With polarity, we are right at the foundation level of existence.

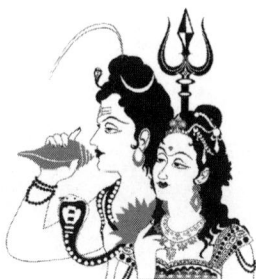

The Sun and the Moon? No.

We have been told that two heavenly bodies represent and reflect the feminine and masculine principles to us. Many might say, "Yes! the Sun and the Moon!" Here I have to take a breath. For this is the problem. This might be one of the reasons why we have become so disconnected from the feminine.

Yes, the Sun magnificently represents the blazing masculine. It's hot, bold dynamism and bright illumination radiate out in all directions with its fiery solar flares exploding out into the world. His constant light and warmth are of continual service to us down here on earth. This is all very masculine principle stuff!

But what of the *feminine*? For millennia, women have looked to the moon for a reflection of who we are. But the moon is no representation of the feminine at all! The moon is infertile, unreceptive and offers no support whatsoever. The moon does not nourish us nor does it nurture or sustain us. Some might say that if the moon were not around at all we would barely miss it. What kind of feminine is *that*?

Don't get me wrong, I love the moon, and I appreciate its effect on the tides and on our monthly and yearly cycles as women and as people. But the moon is not a very good representative of the feminine. There is a much better manifestation of the complex and beautiful feminine principle...

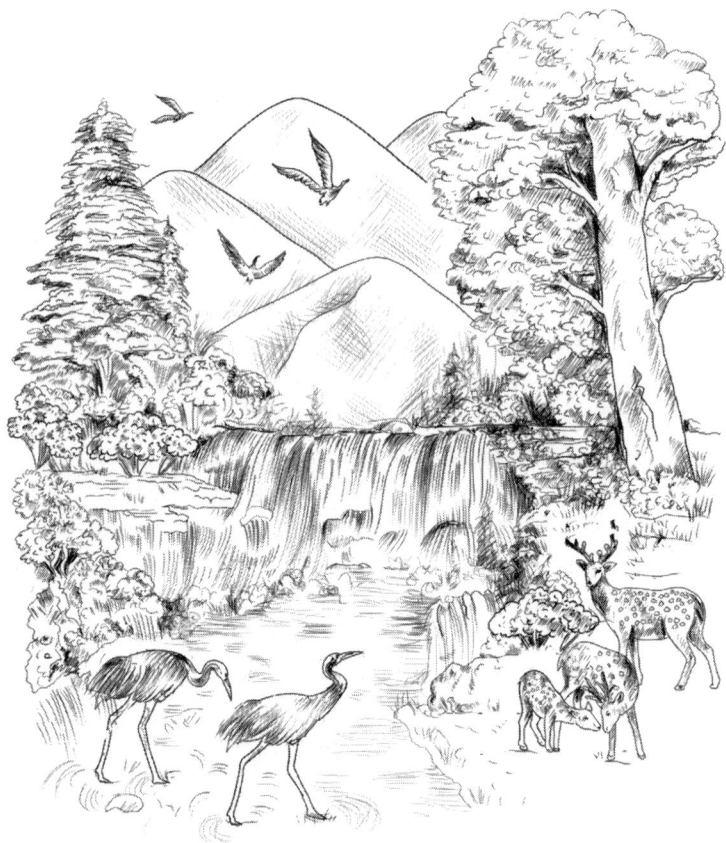

Earth!

The best representation of the feminine principle is actually
right under our feet! Earth has been sustaining us all along! It
is Earth we must connect to and relate with if we are to truly
experience the feminine and truly know ourselves as women...

The Mother of All Mothers

Nature *embraces* us, *sustains* us, *nourishes* us, *supports* us, *holds* us,
energises us and *nurtures* us. Her firm boundaries give us structure
and containment. And, she actually *relates* with us (I'll say more
about this later). She is the mother of all feminine things. Literally.
Everything around us is from her originally. Every product and
item we have on our shelves and in our life is born from her being.

Earth is the inspiration and the Way-shower that humanity
needs in order to remind us what feminine *really* means.

The Earth dimension is packed with delicious goodies!
Unlike the magnificent Sun, Earth does not radiate out so
much. She is much more magnetic, contractive and reflective.
Her force, literally pulls you in. Her field is so strong that it
receives us in and down and holds us to her sweetness to the
extent that it can be difficult to leave...

Complex, Amazing, Wondrous Earth!

Unlike the singular force of the Sun, Earth has a multitude of
different qualities, skills, gifts and energies. Earth is the queen
of variety and brings physical support, nourishment, nurturing,
cleansing, pleasure, joy, communication, healing and everything
manifest. And with Earth we get the shadow too; you never
quite know what you are going to get with Earth as she's full
of surprises. Whereas we always know what to expect from the

25

Sun, only a fool would say that he totally understands Earth! You can stand in one spot and see and feel so many different qualities from just that one place. If you travel 10 miles – you discover more variety still. No day is the same on Earth and no place is the same as any other. And everywhere she is beautiful. Even the ugly places are beautiful.

Earth contains and holds us. She is all structure and boundary. She is the bones of it. She is the banks that guide the river and she is in the bowl that holds the rice. She is the sea bed and the lid on the pot that cooks the porridge. She is the mountain, the desert and the forest. She is both the city and the fields around the village and the spoon that holds the honey.

(If you read aloud the above paragraph to a man who is blessed to have a lady by his side, he may well be smiling at her right now. Because you see, it is we *women* who have no idea how powerful we are; men have always known. They are blown away by our many ways and gifts, not to mention our incredible form.)

Earth produces all the nourishment and resources that we need. Numbers vary, but did you know she has in the region of 60,065 (known) species of tree? Around 230,000 (known) species of flower? And about the same number of herbs? And how many minerals does she have? About 3,000! Known ones that is. Many thousands remain unnamed as yet.

The Amazing Water Element

And then there are her deeply receptive oceans, seas, rivers, streams and brooks... And her freshwater lakes and her puddles. (Even her waters are varied!) About 70% of Earth is covered in water.

Although all of the elements exist on earth, both earth and water are the main elements of the feminine. And these two elements are the most complex and the most mysterious (this

26

never surprises men when I tell them this. Again, they tend to smile and nod).

Water is an incredible element. It is of course incredibly receptive and magnetic and can receive many things. We can see this physically when we have dirty hands and we swish our hands about in bowl of clean water; our hands end up clean and the water ends up dirty! Amazing really and totally taken for granted.

Remembering everything

And in the same way, (and much like women) did you know that water remembers everything? The work of the late Dr Masaru Emoto, talks about this beautifully; how water holds information because it is not just physically receptive but energetically receptive too; to the extent that we can actually programme water to remember stuff! In his book "The Hidden Messages in Water", we can truly see why we women have been dumbfounding men since the beginning of time with an innate ability to remember stuff that they might prefer we forget. (And we wonder why they don't remember things – it's because they are like the Sun – they tend to "burn stuff up" and so get to move on more quickly.)

Birthing universes

Water nurtures us and cleanses us at the same time. Water envelopes us so we can relax. It quenches our thirst and can even sustain life for days even when no food is taken. Running water clears itself too. Huge bodies of water hold and birth whole universes. With very deep water we don't really know what lies there beneath the surface. This has both delighted and terrified us since time began. When frozen, water turns to ice. Add the warmth of the powerful and dynamic Sun, and the ice can't help but melt... and the rivers flow once more and spring returns to the land.

Let us now take a longer look at the marvellous sun and the masculine principle. Through doing this, women can better know the inner masculine and recognise more easily when he is in ascendance. From here, she can make more choices as to whether she does indeed need to temporarily "fire up" the masculine to get something done or soften more into her feminine to access more support from the ground. (Ideally, she would do the latter first.)

The Sun

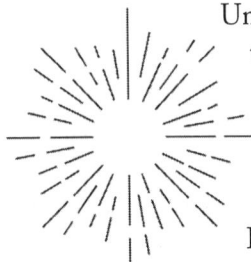

Unlike the complex and beautiful Earth, the Sun's fiery power is very obvious and expanding as he constantly shoots and explodes out his fiery warmth and light. The Sun simply *is* the epitome of light, power, radiance and constancy. He just keeps on going like a dynamo. He is singular in his force. Fire. That's it. One element. Job done. No messing about! If you throw something at him, he burns it up and carries on!

You know where you stand with the Sun. You know what you are going to get. If you don't handle him right, you get burnt. Fire is like that. And his power can provide power for many things. When we see the Sun shining, we might feel warm, awakened and enlivened. His light can gladden our hearts with a spiritual radiance. He brings an incredibly illuminating PRESENCE to our life. With the light on, all is revealed!

And as the Sun shines on Earth? She warms up... she expands... she melts... she opens... unfurls... and she flowers and reflects his light back to him. In spring the sap rises and life begins to birth! In summer, things heat up to such an extent that she pops all her seeds! In winter things are less passionate between these two...

The heat and light of the fire element play a protective role. It has a purifying effect and it also sterilises. The light of fire illuminates, revealing anything that may be lurking in the darkness. Darkness is thus destroyed by light. Fire has a cleansing energy - its flames will clear away anything that is in its way. Many creatures are frightened of fire.

As representatives of the masculine and feminine, the Sun and Earth have been dancing together since the beginning of time. He has never stopped providing her with his powerful warmth and light and she has never stopped responding with unfolding beauty. The more he serves her the more beautiful and reflective she becomes.

The Inner Masculine

As women, it is vital that we know how to utilize the inner masculine so that we are able to protect ourselves successfully by standing our ground, protecting boundaries and by being able to get stuff done! Due to the wonders of polarity and natural law, it is important to have a good understanding of the masculine principle in order to fully understand the polar opposite of the feminine. It is the same with all opposites. If we know "hot" we can better recognise "cool". If we know "up" we can better know "down" and so on. So here I devote a small space to the masculine.

Heat is Masculine, Cool is Feminine

A couple of years ago, I wrote a post in a Divine feminine Facebook group. It was about the Divine masculine within us and how part of this manifestation is anger. I got shot down by a woman who thought I was dismissing *women's* anger and rage. In her rage, she accused me of invalidating women by suggesting that her fire was anything to do with any kind of

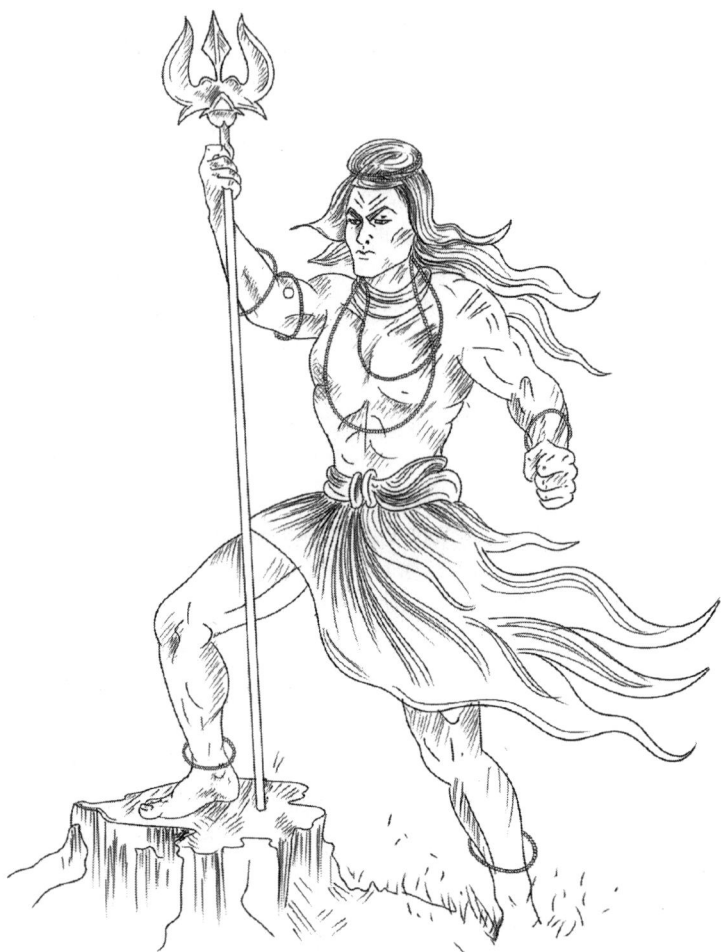

masculine. In her contempt for the masculine she wasn't able to hear that this is a sacred energy within us all. There are many women who feel overwhelmed with outrage due to injustices against the feminine, just as likewise there are many men who have had their masculinity abused (forced enlisting to numerous wars just for a start). Many women have had both the feminine and the masculine beaten down in them and this is true for men too. As I write this, humanity is wounded. But whether we are male or female it is the rise of the Divine feminine that will be helping all and everyone to heal, and it is the rise of the Divine masculine that will be protecting this process and helping us to all forge ahead with it.

In what we might call Western culture, many women have the fire element very strongly expressing within them as drive, ambition and confidence. If this energy is in balance with her core sense of femininity then she will feel joyous and juicy. But if she is using her masculine energy in order to "get ahead" or to compensate for emotional pain, wounding or vulnerability, then there will be a cost, if not just with her mental health, then simply with tiredness or exhaustion.

We might get a sense of how our inner male is in our dreams. In the dream, he might be represented by our current partner, lover, ex-lover or a stranger. He might show up as powerful, handsome and sexy; or he might be wounded, gagged and beaten. We might also see reflections and symbolisms during the day as to how he is.

Building our Inner Masculine

By working to *clarify* our deepest needs and desires we are working with our inner fire element. By then *verbalising* these needs, we are fine-tuning our fire element. This is very empowering and very important. Every time we take courage and express our needs and preferences, we build our fire and confidence, bringing health and

31

balance to our inner masculine energy and to our whole being. This illumination and verbalisation of our needs automatically clarifies our boundaries and protects us. The more we do this and feel how this feels in our body, in our limbs – our arms and thighs especially - and in our whole posture, the more empowered we feel. And the more empowered we feel in our body, the more we are then likely to notice when the opposite is true; so we are more likely to catch that "this doesn't feel right for me" moment and that "I don't want to do this" occasion, and we are more likely to be able to speak up. With this inner protection in place, we are able to relax further into our femininity when needs be. Everything balances up.

Flight, Fight and Freeze

There are times when we feel our inner fiery masculine working at full capacity, and this is when our autonomic nervous system is fully engaged in "flight and fight". Here we feel our masculine fiery power literally "power up" to get us out of danger. But if the event is overwhelming, our fire will "freeze". This is where part of the autonomic system has shut down. The autonomic system is *automatic* and acts out of our conscious control. This is what happens with trauma – our fiery protective system freezes. With loving support after the event, the frozen energy can discharge out (experienced as shaking and/or as grief) and we are free once more and our fire is back online.

Trauma

If support is not available, we end up with trauma. This is where fire becomes water. Frozen energy held in our system. It literally waits there until such time as we feel safe enough to attend to it. Until then, certain events might trigger the freeze response in our nervous system or we might feel the need to flee. We might get triggered into fiery aggressive outbursts or defensive behaviour. Or, the opposite pole could be true, where certain situations trigger collapse, paralysis, depression or feelings of powerlessness and despair. We might find ourselves caught in "victim consciousness" feeling unable to really respond to life's challenges. All of these states, whether our fire is over-expanded or still caught in shut-down and frozen in water, are still an expression of the protective masculine doing its thing. How so? Because all these states protect us from experiencing the overwhelming emotional pain and vulnerability *underneath* the fiery protection. We have to be in a safe enough situation in order to heal this type of wound. So all survival aspects of our personality are an expression of the inner masculine trying to protect us.

With old frozen fire, we can delicately and slowly attend to the overwhelming feelings in manageable bite-sized pieces with a trauma-aware counsellor or therapist. Here, the naturally instinctive reaction to the event can be gradually enabled thus releasing the suppressed fire to be fuelling the system once more. This brings the brain and nervous system back online and re-wires the fire element within us. Even if the trauma therapist doesn't know anything about the fire element per se, trauma-work is directly rebalancing this element because it's directly to do with empowerment and action. This directly engages the masculine principle by helping the fiery energy circuits to reconnect thus enabling empowerment, confidence and freedom.

Healthy Fire

When we focus our fire – direct it into something - things can be achieved; by using our fiery determination we can get to the very end of a project and ensure that we complete it.

Physically, we feel fire in the body as heat when we take direct action of some kind, whether it's getting up and making a cup of tea or the other extreme of experiencing a full "fight and flight" reaction. We feel healthy fire in us when we take an empowered stance, "stand our ground" and hold our gaze.

Digestion

Biologically and psychologically, fire is responsible for our digestion and all metabolism and integration; its fiery action and dynamism enables the digestion of both food *and* experiences. If our fire is blocked in some way then these processes are affected; we may have digestive issues or be disintegrated in some way with food or experiences left undigested. When our fire is in balance on all levels of our being we have that "fire in our belly" that enables all integration of things we experience.

Clear Head, Bright Eyes.

We also know our fire is in fine fettle when we have clear-headedness and decisive thinking. Our intellect is sharp and well-focused. We hear of a "sharp mind" with reference to the knight's sword and the fiery ability to get "straight to the point" and cut through the bull***t. Fire is directed from our eyes with sharp focus and clear vision; and when we have good eye contact, we may even have a "spark" or a "twinkle" in our eye.

Anger

Anger is quite healthy. I distinguish it here from rage and from the fieriness that comes with trapped and suppressed trauma energy which can be violent and explosive. Anger is an appropriate response to injustice or to wrongdoing. We are able to declare with full consciousness, "Hey! That's not okay!" It is vital that we have access to this energy as it is this aspect of the masculine that guards the boundaries that we put in place. For example, we name a boundary like, "only one hour of screen-time for the kids in the evening", but it is the fire element that

guards and protects this boundary and gives us the confidence
to police it. We will tend to feel our solar plexus area "twinge" if
we feel a boundary crossed in some way. If our inner masculine is
very blocked, as children we needed to block our anger and this
might have made us either prone to bitterness or spitefulness or
the opposite pole of super sweet people-pleasing. Both of these
as patterns block the freedom of our inner masculine and the
trapped fire can cause mayhem to our immune system.

Dominance

The masculine; fiery and bright, is naturally dominant.
Illumination simply does dominate. We switch a light on in a dark
room and the space is immediately dominated by the light. It is
the nature of light. As with anything, used without awareness, it
can also cause harm. Used well and with good intention it can
protect and defend. Used by everyone, it is vital when it comes to
achieving certain tasks in order to get them done! If we have to fill
out a form online, we might be dreading it, but we fire ourselves
up, grab our laptop and manfully just get on and do it! Same as
vacuuming – getting hold of the vacuum cleaner and wilfully
pushing it about and getting that job done. Used skilfully by a
man, it can increase polarity in the bedroom.

Competitiveness

Competitiveness too is our fiery masculine energy displaying itself
and this can of course be great fun, but when it's out of control, it's
painful for everyone concerned. This energy is very strong and is of
course fear-based but it is also important not to judge it. I say this
because I believe this competitive energy is a throw-back to the
drive of the sperm that got us all here incarnated in the first place.
The thing is that only one sperm made it, and all the rest died and
so when the masculine competitiveness rears its head, right along
with it comes that fear that if we don't win, "we're screwed". So it's

a powerful energy and needs respect. I believe that competitiveness is vital to achieving many things and if put to good use enables many things to be created and completed.

Protection

Our fiery inner masculine plays a protective role in general. We feel him when we jump to protect and defend another or when we jump to protect and defend our self. We might see the masculine protect physically; with fists or with the legs wanting to flee or kick. Or we might notice ourselves "hardening" (think testosterone!) as our muscles become tense to protect and defend. We might protect ourselves with a "firewall" of aggression and defensiveness. Another way is with avoidance mechanisms; getting stuck in over-thinking and intellectualisation, shutting down, dissociation, or causing a smoke screen or a distraction of some kind as indeed are "word acrobatics" and even ill placed humour. Over-working too, and "driven-ness"; never stopping to surrender into the soft animal body of the feminine. It's all protection. All of these things protect us from feelings and emotions that are lingering in the muddy waters and fecund, peaty ground of the soft feminine body. We all have an integral "bouncer" or bodyguard that is available, to a greater or lesser degree, to help us when we need it.

Enthusiasm

Fire is also responsible for our willingness and *enthusiasm* – that "get up and go" quality that we can call upon if we set our minds to it. It was a revelation to me to discover that enthusiasm is from the verb "to enthuse". A verb is something that we do or not; it is a choice! This is totally in line with my experience of the action and dynamism of the fire element within – we can actually "choose to enthuse" about something. How many times have I *not* done something because I didn't feel enthusiastic about it? Now

I know it's just blocked fire. I can use my breath – as bellows – to bring oxygen to my fire and get on and do what needs to be done.

Determination

Lost your determination? If you push yourself through something you are avoiding, you will feel empowered and if you keep courageously stepping out of your comfort zone you will definitely feel empowered! Doing this very much expands the fire element. Fire and determination are interesting in that we can use determination to expand our inner fire. When using determination to build fire we need to check that the thing we are wanting to do is in alignment with our true purpose. If we use too much determination and leave no space for pleasure, love, fun and relaxation, then "burn-out" can happen in order to wake us up to a healthier way of living.

Confidence

When our fire element is balanced and engaged we feel bright, energised and confident. Many women lack confidence and I find there is a misunderstanding as to why this is so. Some women find that after having children their confidence "goes". But I find that it hasn't gone anywhere. Confidence is a masculine power and women, in becoming mothers, become more *feminine*. We can of course re-connect with our fire and our confidence when we are ready. Bringing our inner fire element into balance by working with empowerment, autonomy and determination brings the masculine principle alive and more confidence comes with it.

Balancing Fire. Inner Marriage

The more balanced our inner fire is, the easier it is to surrender into our femininity. As women, if we over-use our fire, it's a bigger step down into the full lusciousness of our real sexuality. Conversely, if we are not empowered enough and not clear about our needs and desires this equally affects our feminine energy. It's about balance. Healthy expression of fire through clarifying our needs and by taking appropriate action when coupled with surrendering into the many powers of the feminine, enables the divine marriage within us. Here, the Divine Couple; Shakti and Shiva, interconnect and the magic can happen...

Our Feminine Incarnation

In my experience of nearly 30 years of working with children and adults and exploring this subject I have found that the principle we *incarnate as*, generally needs more support than our more hidden inner principle. So if our daughter doesn't like herself and her femininity, or an aspect of it, then this needs a very sensitive response, so that nothing is missed or overlooked. There are moments where the opposite is true - the inner principle will need more support; a little girl may need some help to find her fiery "No!" so that she can protect herself. And the opposite is true where boys need to be shown the magnificence, brilliance and honour of their masculine energy while also having their tears and tenderness supported and being given the chance to prance around in a glittery frock pretending to be the tooth fairy if they so wish. Ideally, neither the feminine nor the masculine is ever rejected in any way.

For many women, the feminine can feel challenging to relax into. This can be for many reasons. For example, if there has been a lot of violence in the family of origin or in the maternal line, receptivity can feel very unsafe. She may have had to numb out, dissociate or "man-up" in some way. This is also true if she is from a family where only masculine attributes were respected. Here the masculine – the archetype of the knight and his fiery protection and solid "armouring" - might feel much safer to stand in. If this sounds familiar to you, just recognizing this is very integrating.

Honouring and having self-compassion for what we needed to do 🌀 as children to fit in with the family we were born into, is the first and vital step on the path of integration and wholeness.

Sexism and Stereotyping

When I talk about the principles, I sometimes hear the terms "stereotype" or "sexist" mentioned. The two things are very different. Essentially, stereotyping and sexism are **limiting** and the principles are **expansive**. Stereotypes and sexism are restrictive and are designed to keep people in boxes and to limit freedom and development. Whereas the principles are the opposite of this. They are *inspiring*. The principles are always *enabling* and are energies for us to aspire *towards* helping us with our development as human beings. Of course, as human beings, we can never totally *become* one of the principles because we need both principles balanced within us for our health.

Diminishing the Feminine

I often see women and girls being deeply disempowered in a way that is quite insidious. It presents as "supportive" but it's subtly disempowering when we are told how the feminine powers of support and nurturing are merely "learned" traits. This diminishes the feminine. Or worse, we might be somehow shown how the watery qualities of softness, receptivity and support are inferior when compared to the fiery qualities of ambition, competition and achievement which tend to be promoted as somehow superior. Here we can see how the feminine powers are suppressed and how over a long period of time, this has impacted on how women and girls experience themselves and how they respond to life on a deep level, with many women feeling disconnected, ungrounded, driven and exhausted - not to mention unwell. (And conversely, with

39

boys and men, the masculine is often spoken of at the same time as the word "toxic", with men's dynamic power now often being dismissed in favour of how nurturing and soft they can be - and this too has had a deep impact on how boys and men experience themselves and how they respond to the world around them.)

With both the masculine and the feminine principles more consciously expressing within us, we might feel more "whole", "together" and "alive". The depth of our strength and the delight of our pleasure and sensual flow of our feminine power is then more consciously part of something bigger. We discover the possibility of truly connecting to a more ultimate experience of our self as Woman. The feminine principle can lead us – show us the way – in a way that our mother might not have been able to show us. It's as if the Goddess Herself is a template we can lean towards.

Bringing it All Together with the Principles

There are two conversations about gender at the moment that seem worlds apart from one another. One conversation is about how men and women are the same and need to be treated the same as each other; where scientists show us how similar we are to one another and gender is seen as fluid and not binary. And then there is another conversation: how men and women are very different from each other, with very different physiology and psychology, and that both genders have clearly different needs; and other scientists show this with equal fervour.

Whatever our experiences and views about femininity and masculinity, the masculine and feminine principles – the two polar forces that make up the whole of creation – are where these conversations meet. You will discover within these pages that both viewpoints are correct; two different perspectives depending on where we set our gaze in any moment. They are not at odds with one another.

The masculine and feminine principles are the real building blocks of creation – they are pre-atomic. These two principles - of opposing forces - are present in everything. that we can sense, perceive, touch, think, see, feel and smell and taste. These forces exist at a more fundamental level than our perception, and underpin anything that we might think ourselves to be. The principles are not antagonistic to our egoic identity but at a more foundational level of existence. All is relevant and all needs to be embraced and brought into the arms of love.

This book is particularly focused on the feminine principle as this is the force that is naturally more hidden and so most misunderstood. Herein I write about the many powers or "ways" of the feminine that together form a very different kind of power to the "empowered woman" we are sold.

The Feminine is Influential

The feminine is receptive and magnetic in nature. It has a "pull" to it. As women, we don't tend to notice this as we are simply busy being this way. But, the masculine knows for sure! The masculine is naturally captivated by the feminine and is hardwired in to serving Her. This makes the feminine incredibly *influential* in the polarity relationship. This power of influence that we have is key to understanding the feminine ways. It is key to understanding the real power that women have in this world even though we are not told this. In fact, we are constantly shown that life only gets exciting when we are using the masculine. This is far from the truth. The truth is far more amazing; that relationships and families generally organise themselves around the desires of the *woman*. *She* sets the standard and the masculine *polishes up* to that standard and this is how everyone develops and grows.

It is *she* who tends to create the lifestyle reality of the family group that she mothers. If she likes packaged food, collecting material possessions and watching TV every evening and all weekend then this will be the lifestyle of her family. Likewise, if she wants to be organic, practice yoga, only do work that inspires her and likes to go for walks in nature on the weekends then this will shape how her family does things.

The Feminine Sets the Standard

She tends to be the one who chooses the things that make up the everyday life that her family experiences. It is *her* health and happiness that are central to the happiness of her family. There is a saying "If mama ain't happy..." The feminine really does shape the world as we know it - but please don't take my word for this. This is what I have seen and see all around me. I cannot un-see it. Do your own explorations and observations and see for yourself. More about this in the Boundaries chapter.

Meanwhile, before we look at these powers individually, there are a couple of things that it is important to know with regard to how we can influence without slipping into manipulation and ego-centred behaviour. For this is where toxic femininity raises its head to be right alongside any toxic masculinity!

Manipulation Versus Influence.

It is through the unmet needs of our inner child that we may get into manipulating. Manipulation is usually done *unconsciously*. If the wounds of our inner child are left to fester, we will find that we get caught in trying to manipulate others and we won't know we are doing it. It is through our own healing and development that we become aware that we are manipulating and trying to control others to get our needs met. After realising that we are doing this, and after working with the much-needed self-compassion, we can choose to tackle life in a new way.

The child manipulates when her needs cannot be met *openly*.
She has to find a way to get what she needs. The parents or carer
are either too busy or too traumatised (or both) to fully support
the child so the child unconsciously finds strategies to get the
energy she needs to survive. While these ways might have been
necessary in our infancy or childhood, it is not so as an adult.
In this now moment, in the safety of an adult body and adult
nervous system, there are more healthy options available and
more healthy ways of finding connection and getting our needs
met. In the now moment we can learn to sense inwardly and dig
deep and explore what we really need, and learn to verbalise this
to people who we know will be able to hear us.

Controlling and Rigid

Controlling behaviour is another way a woman loses her
connection to her influential power. She doesn't mean to do
this. Like manipulation, controlling behaviour stems from
childhood. It's to do with fear. Because of our watery nature, a
woman in particular can easily fall into controlling behaviour
for two reasons, and it's due to the power of polarity.

Control and rigidity are the opposite pole of flow.
Everything exists with its polar opposite. A woman is
naturally flowing, but right there within her is the tendency to
control. We see this controlling water energy in nature when
a large bulk of flowing water simply pushes a person into a
direction that they would rather not go! This happens with
flash flooding. As women, it helps to be very compassionate
with ourselves for our female tendency to control, just as men
need to be compassionate with their tendency to burn (also a
fear-based action). Water is water and fire is fire, and learning
to really utilise these energies and keep them in check and in
balance maybe takes a lifetime.

Bring in the Bowl

For our development as women, now we are in the safety of adulthood, it can help to notice when we are feeling fear. An important question is, "Where is the fear in my body?" Its most often in the chest, solar plexus or belly area with the rest of the body then affected accordingly - with tension often in the back and shoulders, the neck and even the head. Once you have located exactly where the fear is in your body, see how it feels to then bring in the support of your pelvic basin. Sense into your body what happens as you engage with this in-built support within your own system.

Getting therapeutic support of some kind for this particular work can be invaluable.

How Will You Use Your Powers?

In reading this book you will certainly learn how to become more influential and more powerful as a woman. It is therefore important to ask why we want to become more influential and more powerful? What do you want out of it? What would you like to experience?

Setting Your Intention

Here are a few reasons why we might want to be more feminine, more powerful and more influential:
• To be healthier and to feel more alive
• To feel stronger and more joyful
• To attract more wealth
• To know your needs better and be able to sense what you desire
• To know your boundaries
• To help your sweetheart to open their heart more to you, and you to them, increasing polarity and dynamism

• To help your sweetheart become more powerful, confident and successful
• To help bring more romance and more "Wow!" to your life and your relationship
• To feel more wonderful especially in the breast and pelvic area
• To enable sexual ecstasy
• To be able to access more wisdom to support yourself, your husband/partner
• To feel more relaxed and flowing with your children and to enjoy them more
• To inspire your daughter or other's daughters
• To be able to better guide your son or other's sons
• To help change the world for the better

A clear intention brings about a more powerful result. I'm sure you will want to just read on but I encourage you to pause and tune into your heart and belly and see what outcome you would like? When we do this, the universe organises itself around that intention to bring us what we need. Life is like that. Here are some questions below that might be useful:

I would like to become more _____

I would like to create more _____

I would like to feel _____

I would like to heal _____

I would like to be _____

I would like to connect more with _____

Starting with an intention brings about a much more powerful result. So, what would you like to achieve in reading this book? I'm sure you will want to just read on but I encourage you to pause and tune into your heart and belly and see what outcome you would like. When we do this, the universe organises itself around that intention to bring us what we need. Life is like that...

...Let's start with joy! Joy runs the world! Let me show you how...

Chapter 1
Joy

Joy

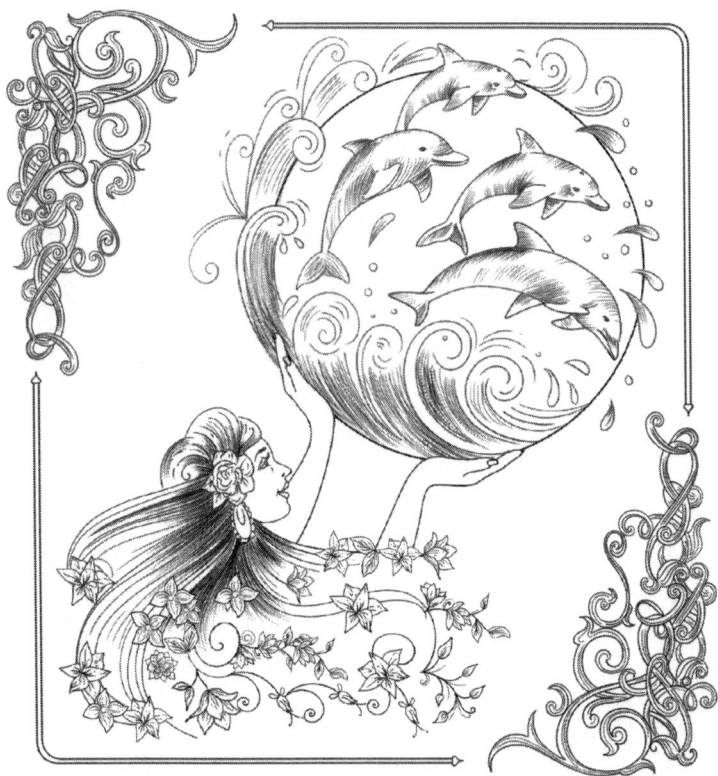

$\mathcal{L}$et's start with joy! Joy runs the world! Let me show you how...

Joy is not an expansive *active* power like running or building a fence – its power is subtle as it influences the context that it's in, and feminine power is like this. We all enjoy joy! Joy is contagious. It lights us up and can raise the spirits of everyone around.

Plants, Flowers and Little Creatures

I see Earth's joy in the form of her plants and flowers and in butterflies and birds and dear little creatures... How do you feel when you see the first flowers of spring? Really feel that for a moment in your body... This is when Earth's joy is waking up after being frozen and frigid all winter. I'm in the UK, so joy shows up as its pure white dainty snowdrops, and then bright mauve bluebells, followed then by the tiny, bright blue forget-me-nots with their vivid yellow centres – all exquisite expressions of joy!

As women, as incarnations of the feminine principle, we have this particular ability to feel and express joy. Joy is very feminine. Men tend to express joy in a very different way. It's quieter. Joy very much expresses from the feminine organ of the heart. If we feel overwhelmed with joy and if we allow ourselves the experience, our heart opens and our tender tears flow from the release.

Women are particularly good at expressing joy, and men tend to be particularly captivated by it - especially if he is romantically involved with her – or would like to be.

Anything for Your Smile

A man will do pretty much anything to see his lady's face light up with joy – especially if he has been the one to cause that. Her joy is his joy. Her smile is his reason for getting out of bed in the morning. Ask any man on a scale of 1 to 10 the importance of his lady's smile and he will say 10 with no hesitation. Ask a woman the importance of her man's smile and you get a more complex answer. His smile is important to her, yes; but not as important as her smile is to him!

The world needs the joy of women. I remember an Amazon review that I read while writing this book. The reviewer was a man and it said, "Well it made the wife smile. Good enough for me!" She may have barely noticed her smile. I suspect she quickly moved on with her work. But he noticed. This is a characteristic of our powers as women, we often don't notice how influential we are. When a man sees his lady in a state of joy, it incentivises him to plan the next thing to make her smile and so on. Men just want to see us happy!

The Masculine Naturally Serves the Feminine

A man is so hard wired into serving the feminine that when his lady is not happy he will automatically think that he has failed. He blames himself for not being able to fix it. We women have no idea that he feels this way as we tend to not think this way ourselves. We women unwittingly shape the world with our joy and have no idea how influential we are in this regard. Please don't take my word for this, experiment and see for yourself!

Men in general become energised when they have been (or perceive themselves to have been) the cause of a woman's joy. But it doesn't matter if he knows her or not. He will hold a door open for her, let her go first in a queue or first into the elevator, and if she responds with a smile, he gets to feel purposeful and more masculine. (Everyone's a winner when polarity is used well.) These are not things he does to diminish her or to patronise her or to be "sexist". Now he *might* be doing that, but if we *assume* this every time a man does something for us then we are totally missing out in the true power of the feminine and the guys are missing out too.

Joy Brings Health to Our Body

Focusing on creating more joy in our life is a particularly healthful thing for a woman to do. It is good for her heart. And it's especially important for women as our sense of self and connection to our sexuality is based on joy. When we fill our life with joyous moments and with the things that bring us joy, it's easier to be grounded and it's easier to be in our body and so feel more pleasure and so on. It also makes us more resilient for when things do go badly. A joy-filled life will keep you energised and able to cope better with its challenges.

The World is Influenced by Joy

Joy makes the world go around in multiple ways. My mind here goes to the multi-million-dollar wedding industry. What is fuelling this massive industry? It's not the guys, that's for sure! It's based on the need for us women to feel joy and the need for our men to see us in a state of joy. The whole creation is led by the feminine. Whether it's the joy of the bride, the bride's mother or the joy of the female guests - the groom and the male guests all get to benefit from seeing how delighted the ladies are! We also know that women in a state of joy are more likely to be loving towards their man, and the guys love this and are of course hopeful...

Whatever is Her Heart's Desire

Men are so influenced by a woman's joy that they will adjust their behaviour if they think this will bring her joy. There is manipulation risk here as with all our powers; if we try and get guys to do certain things or get rid of certain things "so that we can be happy" it doesn't work, but if we influence him it might. For example, a very wealthy man might have seven cars and a palace, but if her heart's desire is to live in a cute little house in the grounds, then this is likely what he will try and create for her. Our power here is such that if a man could not attract a woman through having a plethora of vehicles, several palaces, or an array of guns – he would change his ways for sure. We women have been quietly running the world with joy since Adam and Eve.

Just before I wrote this, a dear friend phoned me. She was annoyed with her husband as he had walked away from her while she was sharing her joy with him. (Golly, was I curious!) She thought he was so rude and she felt really hurt. I asked what was the conversation about. Her energy lifted into joy as she shared how they had been sitting on the sofa together and looking online at these "*wonderful* designer Eco homes with full virtual tours and *everything...*" and before that there were "these *beautiful, intricately,* hand-carved Japanese secateurs for the garden! priced at $500... But they were *beautiful* - such incredible artistry!"

He couldn't afford her smile

I knew immediately what had happened. I told her that I suspected that it was his inner critic that he had walked away from – and not her. He has a very humble job and believed there was no way he could afford to actually bring her the joy of holding those secateurs or having one of those fabulous little Eco houses. It was too painful for him to see her joy and feel powerless to provide her with that which he saw fuelled it. His inner critic probably told him he was "inadequate" and he then probably felt shame.

After I shared my view, my friend's heart melted as she saw him as if for the first time and we ended the call there as she needed to go to be with him...

Nature and Joy in the Home

As women are so like Earth, nature really helps us connect with our joy. Lack of joy can be a real problem in built-up areas that are devoid of nature. Here, house plants can really help! We used to live in a city house but I made the decision, inspired from books I had read in pregnancy, that I was not going to be too precious about the house with kids. Ideally, human kids live outdoors; drawing in the dust and mud and sand and climbing trees and getting into difficulty and out of it again along the way. When we play freely in nature, no one says, "Mind the paintwork!" or "Don't put ya mucky fingers on that tree," or "Mind your muddy boots on that grass." But aesthetics *are* part of what brings me joy, so we found a balance. I did my best to set up the home where kids could freely express joy. One thing I did with no garden was to have a wooden climbing frame built in the living room – slide and all! We had no garden but we did have a generous balcony so we filled it with huge plants and even grew vegetables in the sandpit up there. Joy!

One Joy Every Day

A good practice is to make sure that you really use your power of joy to do at least ONE thing every day that brings you joy. If you are struggling with big issues or if you have a family to support, you will need a lot more than one thing per day. When we have been topped up with things that bring us joy our whole world runs much more smoothly.

Don't skip this next bit. If you do you won't get the results you want. This is where we can use our inner fire of determination to get a piece of paper and make a list and ask a friend to help us. It's not easy, this bit. But it will bring us more into our femininity and our womanhood. Use the energy of rebellion or saboteur to sabotage a family pattern of dismissing self-care and joy. I call this Higher Use of Sabotage.

Deepening Joy

Take a moment right now and have a think about what brings you joy. This can be difficult for us but it's vital to our health as women. Here is a list of things to get you thinking ... and feeling. I highly recommend writing your own list because when we really *need* to experience a full connection to joy and long to make sure we satisfy the need asap – our mind tends to go blank. Here's my list:

- A night time nature walk with a dear friend
- Inviting my neighbour in for a cuppa
- Playing with my cat
- Having a quick go on the slot machine in my local pub
- Having a go on the swings at the park
- Seeing my nieces and my sister
- Running in the summer rain
- Wrapping up in winter and having a walk in nature
- Finding somewhere to go sledging in the snow
- Purchasing a wonderful umbrella
- Summer nature walks making sure I smell the flowers as I go
- Picking wild flowers or finding nature treasures for my table.
- A glass of lemonade in the garden amongst the roses/trees/moss/weeds
- Impromptu baking a cake
- Wearing a favourite piece of jewellery

- Popping to a favourite shop
- Really *seeing* a butterfly – close up.
- Wearing a favourite dress or top or scarf
- Sunbathing naked
- Lying on the lawn
- Skinny-dipping
- A trip to the beach
- Singing while not giving a damn if I'm out of tune
- A game of Hide and Seek
- An impromptu warm bath in the middle of the day
- A nerf gun fight with my son

Exercise: Embodying Joy

To get your experience of joy "planted" in your body, try this:

- Think of something that brings joy. Now imagine yourself with that person/thing or doing that activity and really *feel* the physical sensation of the feeling in your body – especially the area we call the "midline" which is the area from your upper chest down to your lower belly - right down the front of your torso.

- Where does the joy track into your body? There will be a very subtle, felt experience that tells your brain you are feeling joy as opposed to another feeling like fear, for example. Where is the frequency of joy experienced in your body?

- Tracking joy this way means that we have a good strong physical sense of the very real experience of joy that makes it easier to feel.

- Images of the thing you feel joyful about will be in your head for sure, but the actual *feeling* is just that. A feeling and not a thought.

Tip: If you can't tell where the joy is in your body, you might be caught in your intellect. So, while imagining the joyful thing, take your left hand and let it "plonk" onto your midline and trust where it lands. Sometimes the head gets in the way.

Then stay with the real experience of joy and breathe deeply into it.

I do whatever I can to bring more joy into my life. I talk to people I wouldn't normally talk to. I smile a lot. When I buy something from a shop, I have that eye contact with the salesperson or the cashier. I do my best to bring joy and spread joy. Not everyone is able to accept it, but most do.

I want to be open to all experiences that bring me joy. Birds flying overhead in a particular formation, the way my cat sleeps, how it is to see my friend when I open the door to her, the way the leaves on a particular tree change colour in autumn, a house near me that has been beautifully renovated, how I feel when my son comes home from school, how I feel when I see my sweetheart in the car when he's driven to collect me from town and so on. When I spend time in nature, I usually turn off my phone or I don't take it. When I walk and tune in to the nature around me, I actively love her. This brings me joy. Trees and plants give off a lot of energy and I really absorb this into my being and "inhale" this energy – literally. I often say, "I'm off for a walk to inhale some trees." All this brings me joy. ☺

Belongings that Bring Joy

Marie Kondo and her decluttering certainly helps the masses with being more in touch with joy as regards the home. You may feel (even) happier in your home if you notice the things around you that "spark joy" and let go of the things that trigger a heavy feeling. This could be a sense of *obligation* or a heaviness caused by a super ego attack; "Why haven't you read that yet?!" is a super reason to let go of any book that you have not read as soon as you purchased it – which Kondo says is the perfect and only time to read it, otherwise it goes on to the shelf and is added to the other things that you "should" have done, finished, achieved or whatever. "But that was a gift from so and so!" says super ego about that ornament. It may well have been, but does it spark joy? If not, consider letting it go to someone for whom it does. How would it feel to have only belongings around you that bring joy?

The Biggest Killer of Joy: The Super Ego

We all have one of these. Otherwise known as the inner critic, it manifests as self-talk, mind talk and the monkey on your shoulder. This is a protector part of us that stops us enjoying many things. Joy is very much of the heart. It is a delicate thing. If joy wasn't safe to feel when we were a child or if there was an unresolved shock while we were feeling joy, the protector part can come in to make sure we don't feel joy.

So there we are, about to consider a joyous activity and then in comes that voice, "Don't forget you need to do such and such!" or, "Well you can't sit about all day!" (when you haven't sat down once yet)... and so on. Or it can be a dismissing voice like, "What do you want to do that for?!" Or, "How silly!" Either way it's a quiet voice – easy to miss. The voice is located in the head area or over our shoulder or behind our head, but it's always a "neck up" voice rather than the still, small voice of intuition that is experienced very much in the body and is "neck down".

Joy is Delicate

Joy itself is delicate. It's not robust. It is fleeting and open and light and of the heart. And joy is where we may have been hurt as children. Here's a question that women must ask themselves: is it safe *now* to feel more joy? This is a question only we know the answer to. If we are adults and live in a safe enough context with loving enough people then it's probably safe to say that now we can create more joy in our life and bathe in its delicate delights. So we can reassure our frightened protector part – firmly, with words out loud, and say, "Yes, my love... it *is* risky, *all* development is risky, but now we are an adult, it is safe to allow our heart to experience more joy." And then sense into how that feels in your body.

The more we experiment with joy, the more the protector part will quieten about its fears about joy as it will sense that we "have it", and on this issue it is not needed.

Want to find support for feeling more joy? Feel it in your body like in the exercise above. Try it now... Think of something that brings you joy... and then feel where the joy is in your body when you have that sense good and clear; sense down into your pelvic bowl to support that and notice how that feels.

Burn the "To-do" List

My own personal suggestion is to never have a To Do list. *Reminders*, yes. Shopping lists, yes, even a list of vital stuff that must get done today, yes. But long lists of things to achieve? Not helpful. This is the masculine protector energy.

- The masculine likes a goal... being fiery, the masculine is about focusing straight ahead – it likes the future and it loves those goals! The feminine needs more here-and-now pleasure than that. Yes, women like a goal too, for sure, but a long list of things to do won't usually support her. It will support your inner masculine, yes, but not your feminine. This burn-the-To-Do-list idea was fuelled further by my good friend's daughter who said she had heard some research that showed that we get a boost of serotonin (a happy hormone) from either *adding* something to a to-do list OR from actually *achieving* that same thing, but not both. I have personally found this to be true.

Some Joyful Tips

- It helps to keep feminine energy topped up by doing at least one thing a day that brings joy. (Men don't need this as much as women do, as other things charge their masculine energy - like motivation, focus and achievement.) It's all too easy for women to neglect the feeling of joy, and joyful activities tend to be the first thing on the list to go when life gets full. But I see how it's a mistake to do this. Women end up suffering more as do those around them (this is how powerful women are). Doing joyful things each day is vital to our mental and emotional and physical health and enables us to be powerful influencers.
- In challenging times, experiencing something that brings us joy can lift our spirits and enable us to walk more strongly through the challenge. It's not about disconnecting or about dismissing the pain we are in. Neither is it about dishonouring others who may be in pain alongside us. I see it as adding fairy-dust to our present moment so that we are then resourced enough to help our self and help others and do what we are here to do.
- If you have children and they are wrestling with difficulties, after a warm and empathic connection with them, where you have felt their pain and attended to any practical things about their situation, try gently adding joy. It can help to get the timing right as you don't want to interrupt the empathy. But when it's just right, gentle and sweet joy can help to resource and strengthen them and show them that even with all life's struggles, joy can still be found. So turning

a tissue into a funny character or making a little toy do a cheery dance... or suggesting you go find some snowdrops or a squirrel in the garden can enable your young child to digest their difficulty. (Of course, a teenager might prefer pizza or a special film. An older teenage boy might like a task to do to give him a sense of purpose again – with the latter you are the one who would end up feeling more joy. No harm in that!)

- If it feels right, I smile and say hello to passers-by. I chat to staff at my local shop. I smile and say hello to the bin men and I smile and thank the cleaners of the public loos.
- Being a tad rebellious or "childish" can help with bringing more joy. This is because there is a connection between the feminine and the inner child. When is the last time you swung on a swing? Or went skinny dipping? Or rolled down a grassy slope. Just because you can.

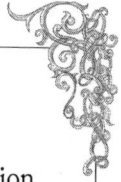

Joy Prayer and Affirmation

You can adjust how you do this prayer and affirmation according to how much fire you need. If you stand and say it out loud with meaning and expression it will fire up your inner masculine so you might end up feeling more empowered and more energised. If you then notice the physical sensations of this in your body, you'll likely have more of a physical experience of empowerment which will help to build your confidence. Or, you might want to do this as a more prayerful practice. You can see what works for you. Either way, the more you do this the more your brain will begin to create new neural pathways around your experience of joy anyway. Isn't this amazing? * Thank you for bestowing me with the delightful gift of joy! * Joy is my nature * I realise joy more and more and feel it deeply in my being * I share the feeling of joy with others more and more * I release the old thoughts and fears that have protected me from joy * I am free now to feel joy * I embrace my joyous nature more and more * I can see that I am a soul incarnate here on earth to experience joy and share it with others * My joy is contagious and many people are influenced by it and feel joy too * I am free to feel more joy! * I reclaim my power to feel joy FLOWING through my body NOW! * The power of joy enlivens and nourishes my soul * I am now connected to the beautiful and delightful feeling of joy! * Yes. Yes. Yes! *

The power of joy enlivens and nourishes my soul * I am now connected to the beautiful and delightful feeling of joy! * Yes. Yes. Yes!...

...Appreciation is how we "switch on" our magnetism and really receive something into our hearts and into our being.

Chapter 2
Appreciation

Appreciation

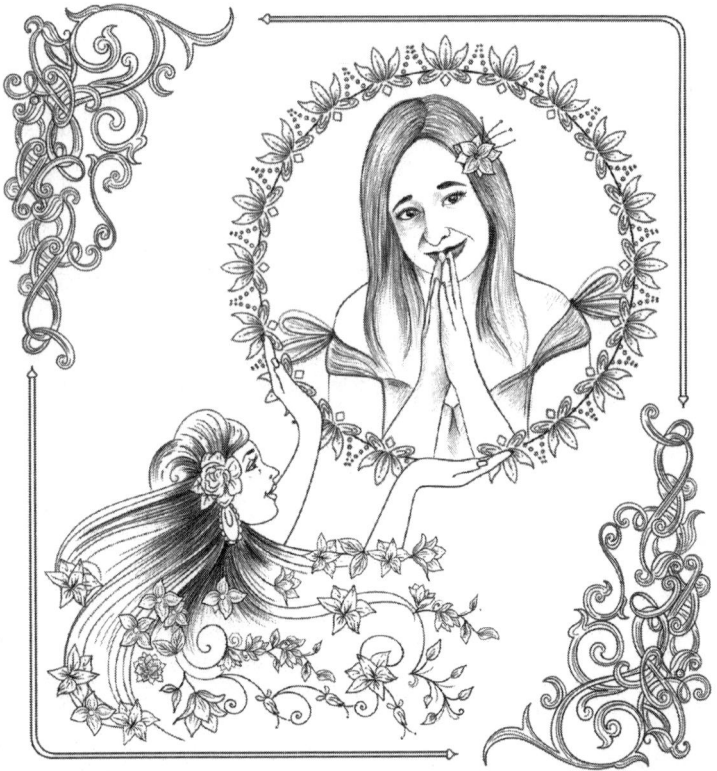

*A*ppreciation is how we "switch on" our magnetism and really receive something into our hearts and into our being.

Whether we would like to attract more wealth, a particular item, more attention from our partner or if we'd like to create a New Earth, then starting with appreciation for this very thing enables it. Literally imagining this thing or this reality in our very mind right now and feeling appreciation for it is how we manifest it.

Appreciation Creates More Magnetism

This "sending out" of appreciation creates the opposite effect of energy "coming back" to us. This movement is taught by those who teach wealth creation as it's known that appreciation, as well as gratitude, is the path on which wealth and energy flows towards us. It doesn't matter whether you are male or female, using the magnetism of the feminine force is what opens us up to receive that which we would like.

Appreciation changes the way the universe responds to us as it engages our innate magnetism. In doing this it can bring about a shift in the relationship that we have with the people around us. Switching to appreciation can change the dynamic of even the trickiest relationship, no matter how awkward things are – especially if the other person is a man.

Feel It in Your body

As you appreciate things and people in your life, how do you experience this in your body? I notice as I feel appreciation, I can feel the gravity in my body "open". There is a softening in my heart. As I continue and keep observing the sensations in my body, I then notice a feeling of pleasure even in my yoni as my whole feminine nature wants to envelop that which is on its way to me. I ground and anchor this energy, this experience, at my feet and find my breath deepens.

Appreciation Ignites Our Man

When a woman practices appreciation in her relationship with her man, he will be particularly responsive to it. If we verbalise our appreciation and gratitude and communicate our pleasure when our man has done something for us, their naturally expansive masculine energy is ignited on a fundamental level and they are then many times more likely to want to do that thing again. This is pure polarity in action! Appreciation has a positive effect on women too – if we don't feel appreciated, it hurts! Men, however, are particularly responsive to appreciation and gratitude as their whole being can feel as if it is being received and accepted and this charges their masculine energy as it gives them a sense of purpose and ambition.

Earth herself is very appreciative of the way we attend to her and of our affection towards her. In our culture we tend to be switched off to this – but many can feel it! Some may see Earth as something we have to take care of – a burden even. But this is just because our perception of her appreciation has not been realised yet. We are not really in *relationship* with her. Earth is seen as an "it", and we may experience ourselves as walking about on "it". But this is not actually the case at all, and those that really spend time in nature connecting with her consciousness know this deeply.

Nature as She and not "It"

Have you tried actually interacting with nature as if it were a "she"? We might tenderly touch a plant or tree, or even verbalise how beautiful they are. Or we might appreciate a pond or lake and notice how it responds. Sounds a bit cuckoo I know, but until we have had a go at sensing this kind of thing and observed the results, we might be dismissing something that could actually help us. While perceiving Earth's response to our actions, it helps to trust what our imagination sees. I believe the imagination (our ability to see images) is deliberately undervalued in our culture because it's a very powerful ability. I experience our imagination as a type of bridge or communication between us and the elemental world and also to the other dimensions.

Letting Go into Appreciation

Women often have a hard time accepting appreciation from others. Her own magnetism will have her quickly looking inward and noticing all her fault-lines and wonky mountains and then she might bat the appreciation or gratitude away. "Oh, it's just a simple recipe." "Oh, this is an old dress I've worn for years!" She might even become defensive. Many women can find it almost too painful to be appreciated. Every time we are appreciated it helps to let-go a little inside and take a breath… and say, "Thank you, that's really kind."

Men Only Get Appreciation from Women

Whereas women may often attempt to appreciate each other, men don't tend to get appreciation from other men. Men often tease and even insult each other and relate in a very different way. If men work on their inner feminine by developing their emotional life they might find it easier to appreciate each other. With the dissolution of the tribe – who would cheer and welcome the men home from the hunt – this now leaves men quite dependent on only their women to offer appreciation to them in order to help keep them motivated. If men were cars, appreciation would be their fuel. This is one reason why men suffer the way they do if they are unemployed or if they feel purposeless – they are then less likely to be appreciated and this compounds things.

The Masculine Gives, the Feminine Receives

Just as the Sun serves Earth, the masculine is hard-wired into serving the feminine and the feminine is hard-wired into receiving his services and gifts. This is the nature of polarity and both get energy from this relationship. Appreciation for male's natural ability to serve can really heat things up within a relationship. I believe this is what makes it really difficult to find a suitable gift for a man. We never know what to give him do we? However, appreciation and good food is a great gift to give a man.

Mr Hot Guy

I'm reminded of a very handsome silver-haired hunky guy who waited very gallantly for me to pass him on a narrow strip of footpath in central Cambridge. The narrow section was long because of building works, so I had a bit to walk and he had a bit to wait while watching. But I noticed immediately his interest in me. This would have just been an ordinary moment if I hadn't found *him* so hot! This is key. Because of *my* attraction to Mr Hot Guy, my appreciation back towards him had a powerful force to it and he felt it and it supercharged the exchange. It made him *beam*, expand and radiate towards me and the charge between us increased even more! He was beaming and I was melting, and walking past him was like WOW! I think we both felt appreciation ☺

The thing to get here is that my appreciation of him is what got this dynamic charged up. If I'd have just thanked him politely, the charge wouldn't have been so high. But *my* appreciation back towards him is what made the event what it was. We women are the ones with the power here. This same dynamic can be happening with same-sex folks too.

As with all the feminine powers, women are not as aware of their power of appreciation as much as men are. Ask any man how much he needs appreciation from his lady and he might open up to you and you might learn something from him.

Gifts from Him

It's easy for us to get caught in the wounds of our inner child with regard to appreciation. When a child is given a gift, whether it's a gift-wrapped item or an action done with intention, a young child will only appreciate that gift or result if she approves of the actual thing that is given. She doesn't understand about *intention* yet. What *adults* do is appreciate the *intention* and heart-felt energy *behind* a gift or action even if that gift or the outcome is not quite to our liking.

Many male/female couples get caught out here. Many men find themselves withdrawn and crestfallen when their attempts to serve their lady go unappreciated. Men are so wired for giving that when their gifts are declined this can feel like a deep rejection and they will feel additionally foolish for feeling this way. Many women, especially those who had an "ill-attuned" mother who did not meet their child's needs, find themselves triggered into childhood anger and disappointment as "yet again" we haven't been given what we really wanted or the thing hasn't been done exactly how we would have liked. If we haven't been able to fully process these old, deep feelings of disappointment, sorrow, fear and rage, this will prevent us from feeling appreciation when our man is actually doing his best. If our nervous system is triggered, the charge of the old triggered feelings will be dominating our body in the present moment and we will feel fragmented and in great pain in that moment. We will be in our childhood trauma place and quite unable to feel appreciation for his efforts. Here, choosing to come from a place of self-compassion for how we feel can help us to integrate these old feelings.

Housework, Appreciation and Standards

Housekeeping is where resentments can really build-up in the polarity relationship. Here's the thing: if a woman and her man live together, the home is her nest. It might be his castle but it's her nest and he is in her nest! He is a lucky guy and he knows it. If he lived alone in the castle, the place might not be as tidy - and for some men this is putting it mildly. (I am actually messier than my sweetheart, but in other areas my standards are definitely higher!)

With the odd exception, if this same man cleans the worktops badly, what this is *actually* showing us is how he wants to please his lady and make her happy. If there was some passive-aggressive stuff going on here, he's more likely to avoid doing it altogether. Women often project onto men because of the way that *we* behave and think as women.

We Project Our Thoughts onto Our Man

For example, a woman may do a slap-dash job just because she is very busy but she might also do a bad job if she wasn't conscious of how angry she felt. Men rarely do this as their fire is so "up front" and visible. So, we might project onto our man that he is being passive-aggressive or resentful, and he may well be, but there is also a good chance he isn't being this way.

We women tend to be much more underhand with our anger and resentments (think deep water hiding stuff) whereas men tend to be more obvious with it (think fire). Passive aggressive behaviour is of course a thing. Look for other signs if you think your man is doing this and consider giving him some loving and honest reflection so that he can get the feedback to develop. For you; why might he be angry with you? Do you make it easy for him to be honest with you about how he feels?

Women Set the Standard

Women set the standard in a relationship and men polish up to those standards. Most men, if left to their devices, would live in a mess or the cleaning would be left. In a nutshell, more often than not, if he is cleaning the work surfaces or doing any other stuff around the home – he's doing it for you or because he is influenced by you.

Men and women living together *is* a challenge. I think tribally, women live together and share the chores and inherently sense or know what needs doing. The guys might do their own thing and flit in-and-out focusing on other things, or they lie about and charge up their in-built batteries ready for some high-powered action like hunting, building or harvesting.

Marshall Rosenburg, the creator and developer of Nonviolent Communication, says that there are two sorts of people in this world - Tidies and Untidies - and they always seem to end up living together! Using appreciation is a powerful way of resolving this issue and it works powerfully indeed!

When He Gets It *Really* Right

If you appreciate your man when he *does* leave the worksurface spotless, he is very likely to do it again. He'll do it just to get the appreciation and see you joyful, as this is what makes him tick. This is also more likely if you have been very clear with him as to why you are appreciating him. "Oh wow you even did under the toaster! Fabulous darling!" Men don't make connections in the way women do, so make sure he knows *why* you are delighted.

You Are Not His Mother

Some women may think it's patronising to speak to men in this way. There is a fear that treating men in this manner is treating them as a child, therefore making him more like one. Two things here: the feminine tends to be wiser and more nurturing and less likely to behave irresponsibly. Men, being so fiery, simply do tend to behave rashly or irresponsibly sometimes and can often seem childish - the fire element is like that – it can't help shooting out sparks or solar flares spontaneously and people *do* get hurt. Men simply do need some help with boundaries around this and they are the first to admit it. This is why men simply tend to do better in life with a good woman by their side. Secondly, but maybe most importantly, just because he is behaving as a child, does not automatically make you his mother. This is "over-connecting" – a thing that women tend to do – connecting two things together that aren't connected and then getting upset about it. However, there is a similarity between the masculine and children, in that both need clear boundaries and clear goals! Men and kids both need standards to polish-up to. Both men and kids then need additional appreciation and acknowledgement when they have achieved those goals. The feminine doesn't tend to need this to the same extent, or rather, she needs other things more – such as adoration, pleasure, to feel joy, to laugh, to stroke a kitten...

Appreciation Makes Him More Manly

Having said all this, a woman will indeed resent her man if he spends all his time in child mode. If she is a mother, she will be super sensitive to this and her sexual desire will go as flat as a pancake. She doesn't need an extra kid. She needs a *man* to show up, get stuff done and make her swoon. A woman may indeed resent having to speak skilfully to her man by expressing her desires in order for him to find his own heroism with heroic action; "God, I can't be bothered to treat him with kid gloves! I just want him to get on and do stuff!" Yes, men do need to get stuff done, for sure, but men are such completely different creatures to women and we have not been taught how to respond to this. But when we get it right with our man, the rewards are many!

The Masculine is Fuelled by Appreciation

Men think completely differently to women. Men become ignited by appreciation. It makes him feel good and it makes him want to serve more. I have seen this time and time again. Women like to feel good by being treated a certain way; and men do too. Appreciation in *particular* makes men feel good and we women are highly influential with this.

It's not about appreciating your man in order to make him work even harder to fund another bathroom re-fit that you don't really need and that doesn't really serve Earth. This is manipulation. But if your old bathroom needs some new taps, new plugs and a shower that works, then appreciating him will surely *motivate* him in a way that he might be more *likely* to do stuff around the house. If he does, he would get a testosterone boost from achieving all that and you would be more likely to be worshipped like a Goddess when he makes love to you. Everyone's a winner here - even Mother Earth.

If you have a man in your life, due to the incredible power of the polarity relationship, notice the impact your special appreciation has on his heart and his fire. Practice giving appreciation to those around you more – men and women - and you will see how influential you are. But with your man especially, it's about building the energy, building love and building a level of amazing charge between you and the masculine and creating a better life and a better world. Let's raise the vibe and appreciate frequently!

Some Appreciation Tips

- I find a useful thing to do is tell my man something every day that I appreciate about him (I'm just going to do this now as I haven't done it for a few days!)
- If you have a brother or father or son, we can deepen our connection with him by telling him what we appreciate about him. We can do this even if the person has passed on.
- I also express appreciation to teachers at the local school, the staff in the corner shop and to call centre staff who answer my call when I'm sure they'd rather be less enslaved to the system they find themselves in.
- I always notice how it feels in my body when I have appreciated someone. This generally helps with embodiment and builds presence and pleasure.
- Men tend not to make as many connections as women do. So when I appreciate my man or my son, I will often say precisely *how* they have helped me; "Thank you so much for doing that my love as it means I can get on with editing my book much more quickly now." When we do this, it helps the masculine see exactly how they have served us, and it gives them more of a sense of purpose. It's very motivating.
- It's useful to remember that just because we are appreciating

74

our man for doing stuff around the house, that does not mean that we are suggesting that he is doing it for us "because it is our responsibility to hold the housework and not his". If a man is doing housework it is more often the case that he *is* either doing it for his woman or to actually polish up to the standard that she sets – to be a better man. If you have one of those men that is very tidy and house-proud, then every time you appreciate this about him he will feel even more motivated to be that way. It will feel affirming to him and he will then more likely adore you more. Win/win.

- Another useful exercise is to appreciate our body. Many years ago, I was learning holistic anatomy and physiology and the teacher invited us to close our eyes and send love and appreciation to our heart – the actual organ. We did this for a while and then shared what we had noticed. I was quite surprised by what I noticed! I had an image of my blood having been kind of "lit up" by my love and appreciation as it flowed away from my heart. And so, as it travelled further round my body, my whole circulatory system ended up being lit up!

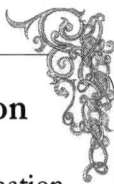

Appreciation Prayer and Affirmation

You can adjust how you do this prayer and affirmation according to how much power and fire you want to create within yourself (see Joy Prayer and Affirmation). * Thank you for bestowing me with the wondrous gift of appreciation! * I appreciate my own gifts and skills that grow in strength every day * I appreciate my loved ones and the little things they do and I notice this more and more * I appreciate my body and all its curves and creases and how it is a temple to my soul and spirit and has enabled me to be here in this world * I practice the power of appreciation more and more in my life and in my day * The power of my appreciation is so strong and I can feel mine and others' spirits lift * I find more and more things to appreciate in my life! * I honour that I am a soul incarnate here on Earth to appreciate all of life around me * I create more and more things in my life that I can appreciate * I build many friendships and connections and I appreciate them all * I appreciate the Great Power that has enabled me to be here alive at this time *

I create more and more things in my life that I can appreciate * I build many friendships and connections and I appreciate them all * I appreciate the Great Power that has enabled me to be here alive at this time *...

...Hey sister! You are as strong as a deep river flowing to the sea! Did you know this? As a woman you are endowed with this power for sure!

Chapter 3
Strength

Strength

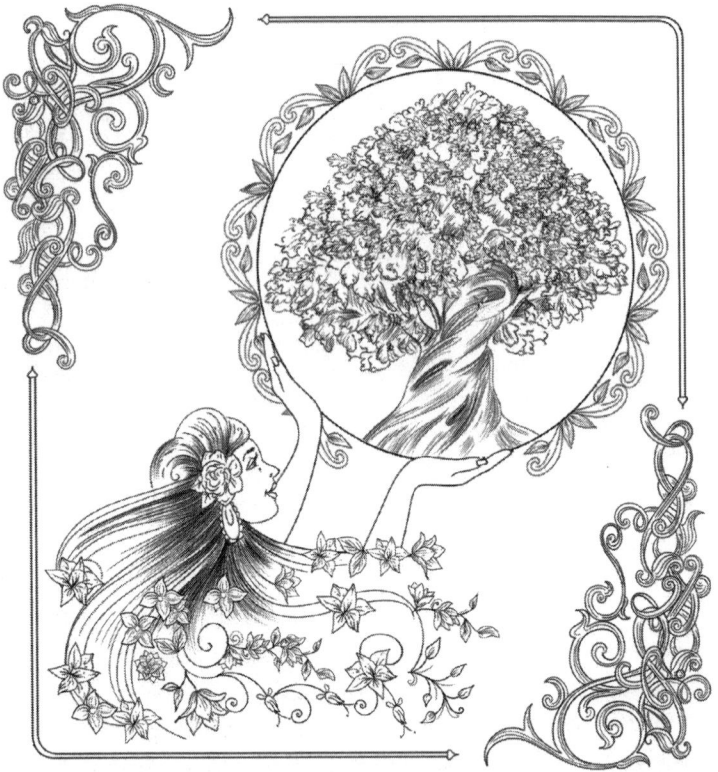

*H*ey sister! You are as strong as a deep river flowing to the sea! Did you know this? As a woman you are endowed with this power for sure!

When I was writing this chapter, it was early spring in 2019. The footpaths in my village had been tarmacked in the autumn of 2018. But what did I see here? The most delicate dandelion shoots... pushing upwards... right up through the tarmac! Leaves so delicate that if I'd touched them I might have bruised them and yet these tiny, tender shoots were having the silent strength of a cosmic giant to push upwards through this horrid tarmac!

How so? Such is the strength of the feminine! The feminine has a delicacy, yes, but a strength that is paradoxically inherent in all her creations; her leaves, her flowers, her ants... the ability to sustain and to survive; to stretch and to endure...

Strength or Power

I distinguish "Strength" from "Power". Feminine strength is a very different force to that of the masculine quality of fiery, dynamic power. When my clients experience strength and really *feel* this energy in their body it is described as a "solid", "strong all over" or "weighted" experience. These descriptions tend to be accompanied by a sense of "calmness", or even "quiet peace". We are talking more about the calm strength of the mighty oak than the expansive power of the fire within the blacksmith's forge, which tends to feel more energising, dynamic and empowering.

Strength compared to power is more a centripetal, "inward" and compacting force. Think of the strength of a diamond. Strength can take a lot of pressure! If I see a woman juggling a lot or having to deal with a lot of stress, I often say, "Oh thank goodness you are a woman so you have the strength to deal with all this!"

She is Queen

My local garage has grown and grown from a small two-man outfit to a large business employing many staff. The owner, Steve, employed Becca a few years ago as the receptionist. I have been going there for many years now and what I see is Becca running the show and I suspect that Steve knows this! Her feminine strength means she can deal with much pressure. She is always doing several things at once; holding many things in her feminine energy. Like a fruit bowl holds many fruits, the feminine holds many things too. She is strong like that. Throughout the day, she is waiting for parts to arrive from several different suppliers, while helping customers and suppliers on the phone and dealing with customers in the reception area. But everything flows. She has now brought in comfy sofas and plants for customers to wait in a nurturing environment. Off she pops to the workshop with a mechanic to see exactly what he means by a "such and such" part that he needs and back she comes to order it, while politely dealing with all the customers on the way and while the phone is ringing. Multi-tasking to its extreme, she is queen of that place. The mechanics feel her support and her strength. It's tangible. The business is booming.

Strength is Solid <u>and</u> Flexible

The mighty energy of Earth is very *solid*. There she is... gigantic, colossal and totally "there". If you push against her – she meets that in equal measure; she makes a corresponding push against you - to meet you. If you try it now – by pushing your foot into the ground or by pushing into Earth... can you feel her solid strength? She is SO ROBUST! If you jump up and down on her, stamp on her, push against her - she just *meets* that.

Nothing budges her.

The flexibility of the water element is strong in a different way to solid earth. The strength is in the flow and in the flexibility that comes with that. A little drop of water when repeatedly dripping can wear a hole into a stone. A stream of water can persist and make its way down to the sea, flowing over obstacles, taking all sorts with it, building momentum. Water from a leaking pipe can trickle its way out and down, and if allowed, can bring a house to collapse! And the sea... the strength in those big waves! You are like this. As women we are like Earth and her great seas and oceans.

The Inner Strength of the Feminine

I have heard men acknowledge the strength of their women. I have heard them speak of women's ability to "go to certain places emotionally" where they themselves cannot easily go – or where they may more immediately resist going. In this regard, I've heard many men say "I'm not strong enough to do that." Men admire the emotional strength of women.

Women seem to have the ability to admit things about themselves and feel stronger having done so. We tend to have more ability to self-reflect and to take responsibility for difficult situations that we find ourselves in. We tend to find it easier to grieve. For some men, grief feels worse than dying... he'd rather stay upright... shining forth, proud like the Sun and this feels more healthful to him.

The Inner Work of the Feminine

Women, being so feminine and centripetal, like gravity, are naturally predisposed to inner work, self-discovery, personal growth and healing. I remember an old male friend of mine,

who was honouring his wife's therapy journey, saying that
he didn't feel strong enough to do it. He thought she was so
strong to keep querying and allowing and letting go; and what
an amazingly honouring man to respect her like this.

But so often I hear a woman exclaiming about her man,
"Why must I be the one to always do all the development and
growth work?!" I can relate, but...

Women Lead the Way in this Realm

As a representative of the feminine principle, women are
naturally magnetic. This is a very strong energy, like a diamond.
And a diamond has gone through a long process to become
what it is. Women naturally find it easier to turn inwards; to look
inwards and self-reflect – as we are like water and earth. Men
being so masculine are naturally more centrifugal – like fire – and
so tend to find it easier to look away from themselves and this is
great with their inner capacity for service but more challenging
for them to heal emotionally and come into their hearts. It is our
capacity to turn inwards coupled with our emotional strength that
literally *shows* them how to do this. Women's emotional courage
and capacity to "go there" emotionally reflects their man's inner
feminine back to him and shows him how to be in his heart and
escape from the trap of his head.

Our magnetism and strength mean that it does tend to be
easier for us to step into a healing relationship with our selves
– with our inner little one – the wounded child – and perhaps
also with a therapist, healer or counsellor, to accomplish
this further. Our man will tend to be influenced by our
development. I have seen this time and time again. (I also have
had male clients who have led the way in their relationship as
regards healing because they have such a strong inner feminine;
but this is more unusual, I find.)

Development Takes Strength

Because we women are an incarnation of the feminine principle it is particularly easy for us to develop and change. Nature is constantly developing and changing and women are too. Not just through maiden, mother and crone but even within these stages too. Our capacity to change makes us naturally strong. I remember an elderly man saying that in his long marriage to his wife he had seen her become about six different women and he saw his job as one to support these different phases. Men often find change more challenging. Their masculine fiery energy is more about constancy and staying the course. Men are inextricably drawn to women, as women help men to develop by setting a higher standard and by bringing him into his heart.

Some men might feel inadequate around women. I see this as part of the masculine wound – where, through lack of warm fathering, leadership and mentoring, they haven't been able to fully step into their manhood yet. True manhood is brilliantly awesome and radiantly warm and does not know envy of women as he knows deep in his being that both the masculine and the feminine are wondrous.

When we have full connection to the physical power of strength within us, we tend to feel the felt-sense of this all over our body and down into our legs and feet. We may feel as if we are "rooted to the spot". Not in a frozen unpleasant way, but in a strong and flexible way. Mother Earth IS SO STRONG! Her strength and her resilience are ours to feel and sense into.

The Strength of Mothers

I remember my father mentioning a family in the village. They were a large family with many children and he described the woman as a cheerful and welcoming woman who had willingly

invited him into her home as he called by to return something.
Even though her hands were obviously full with the needs of
many - with her children all running around her, and to and
from her - in the midst of all this she made my father a cup of
tea and offered him some homemade cake. She sat and chatted
with him with the children carrying on as children are prone
to do. This is the kind of strength we women have access to.
I'm not saying a man would not do this. He might indeed,
but if Mr Neighbour had invited my father in, rather than
Mrs Neighbour, I suspect it would perhaps have been a very
different afternoon, and I have a feeling my father wouldn't
have felt so welcomed and loved.

The Strength of Childbirth

Men have long admired the strength of women to give
birth to their babies. The 3-day labour, the movement of the
pelvic bones, the flexibility of the feminine body, the going
without food for a long period of time and the management
and transcendence of the pain. The medicalisation of birth
has meant that many women have been and continue to
be prevented from experiencing this level of power within
themselves. Midwifery skills appear to be narrowing but
Doulas (birth assistants and Wise Women trained to support
women to birth their babies) are becoming more and more
popular as women want to experience the full depth of their
power in the birthing process.

Earth Energy Strengthens Us

Strength is quite a deep and continuous force. Strength is
perhaps the "sea-bed" of the feminine powers. By rooting
deeply into Mother Earth and feeling her energy come right

up into our body through our feet and legs, charging our womb and our ovaries, we are truly strengthened. It doesn't matter what is going on for us; how much pain we are in and it doesn't matter what we have done and how ill our behaviour. Earth is there for us. She's never conditional and she never rejects or abandons us. Her strength and love for us never wane. It's important for men to tune into Earth energy as well, to strengthen them. I have found that there is not quite so much resonance between men and the Earth plane as much as between the Earth plane and women. I have found that men tend to be much better at meditating as they can silence their mental chatter more easily and tend to focus more effectively.

Soft Is Strong

Very wounded women can feel quite "hard" or "brittle". This can be because they have had to rely heavily on the inner masculine within themselves to protect them and as they have had to "man up". In doing this, many women lose connection to the delights of the feminine. A woman does gain power here but she loses her strength. She might even feel weak. Tuning into the strength of Earth and really feeling her support can help here. Time and healing hands may bring the waters of the healing rivers to wash through her psyche and leave her strong and flexible and tender once more.

"Grow a Vagina"

Kim Anami, in teaching her vaginal Kung Fu quotes a woman who was querying the saying "grow some balls" with regard to those times when we need to achieve something or be brave. As the woman she quotes rightly says, testicles are actually incredibly fragile and very delicate but the vagina by comparison can "take some real pounding" and is actually incredibly strong! Do life with full awareness of your amazing vagina and let her incredible elasticity and flexibility bring strength to all you do.

It is interesting to note that the otters, according to Native American Medicine, are the medicine for femininity and the otter is so very flexible! We are able to stop our work and attend to a friend in need or change tack to do something else that needs attending to.

So dear sister, feel the beautiful and strong Earth under you. She is part of you and you are part of her. How does this feel? Notice. How does this feel in your body? You might want to say it out loud or write it down as this helps to programme your brain and nervous system with this feminine power of strength.

You can work with building your connection to this strength that you naturally have resonance with. You can build it.

Strength Exercise

This is a very specific exercise that, like meditation, might not "click" for you straight away. For some of us can get so disconnected from Earth that to reconnect becomes a process... a journey. When I am with people in my therapy room, I am able to guide them to this. Essentially, I am inviting you to connect with the magnetism of Mother Earth. When fully engaged with her field there is a subtle, "heavy" feeling of weighted strength.

1. Sit in a chair with your feet placed flat on the floor. You might want to lean back in the chair to enable relaxation.

2. Deeply sense into your feet on the ground, and when you have done this, next sense into your sitting bones. This might be tricky if your chair is soft but quite possible.

3. Now feel the chair under your bottom and under the back of your legs and at your back.

4. Back to your feet now and take a few breaths and r-e-l-a-x...

5. Breathing deeply into your lower belly now. Feel your lower belly shrink as you exhale... And then feel your belly expanding as you inhale - first filling up the lower belly *before* you fill up the chest cavity. Do this a few times.

6. Feel how Mother Earth, in the form of the chair and the floor – and in all the "things" around us – all made of her energy – is ***present*** and isn't going anywhere. Feel her *solidity*. Sense into how she is pushing up to meet you with perfectly equal counter-resistance.

7. Notice how if you push your feet a little into the floor how she pushes back with equal measure; if she pushed back with more force your feet would rise upwards. Any less and your feet would sink downwards. But they don't. Because she always gets it right. She always gets the pressure perfect. Perfect attunement. She knows just how much pressure to "meet" your very being. Stay with this for a while simply sensing and observing how this experience is in your body. How does this feel?

8. Now sense into Earth's massive body. The *hugeness* of Earth... her colossal size. Unfathomable strength.

9. Sense this strength in *your* body.

10. Her strength is your strength. If you have connected, you will feel this subtle, weighted, heavy, strong feeling. Do not be concerned if you can't sense this yet. Keep breathing and sensing...

11. If you can feel it, next, breathe this strength energy into your womb. Just breathe deeply and imagine it going there. The womb is so receptive and containing that it can hold Earth's nourishing energy and this strengthens us.

The more often you do this, the stronger you will feel and the more able you will be to cope with life's challenges.

Men and boys can do this too! Imagine storing the energy in the belly or even the testes. It is deeply strengthening and brings a sense of deep inner support.

Our Strength Helps Us Process Feelings

The exercise above is useful to do every day as it brings detachment from feelings that we might otherwise be over-identified with. It's good to do alongside what I call *astute observation* as it enables feelings to be observed... to let-go and ground-out. Our connection with Mother Earth takes the drama out of an emotion and halts the story of it that might fuel it and over expand it. Doing this exercise enables us to stay with our own present moment no matter how challenging it is. This exercise can actually help us to process and transmute many feelings. It stabilises the nervous system too.

Men can become stronger psychologically by finding a safe place to come into their body and their feelings. Here their inner feminine can bring more flow, wisdom and strength into their masculine fiery psyche.

Grieving Makes Us Stronger

Sometimes blocked or suppressed feelings or emotions are effectively *in the way* of our connection to the ground and to strength. We have to go *through* the water (emotions) to get reconnected to the solid stuff (strength/earth/grounding). Either way, grounding at the feet and at your sitting bones or sensing down into the support of all the bones in our pelvic basin helps contain and give *boundary* to what is going on and so keeps things at a manageable pace.

Grounding with Your Inner Child

When we ground ourselves, we can change history and mess with time. If, when we ground, we include our inner child into our heart as we do this, we effectively sit with our little self on our knee. Here then, we literally re-stitch the tapestry of our childhood. We are adding strength in the now moment where strength was missing in the past. And we can whisper to the space, knowing in our bones that she can hear us, "Hey sweetie... I'm your adult self... let's sit together... let's ground awhile and feel Earth's strength in us."

Some Strength Tips

- When I find there is a lot going on and I doubt my ability to cope, I say to myself, "I am a woman, so I am naturally strong."
- Sometimes I do the strength exercise as a little meditation.
- If I find myself becoming rigid and inflexible, I remind myself to breathe and bend and sway like a great oak. Strength is flexible.
- If someone is new to this work and is asking me, "But what *is* the feminine?" Or, "How do I stop using the masculine all the time?" I get them to do the Strength exercise. It's often a game-changer.

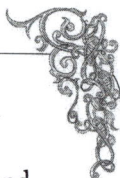

Strength Prayer and Affirmation

You can adjust how you express this prayer and affirmation according to how much fire you want to create. (See Joy Prayer and Affirmation.) * Thank you for bestowing me with the wondrous gift of *strength* * I am **so strong** * I feel this strength in my body and I allow it to permeate my being! * I re-claim my strength! * I allow my strength * More and more I embody the power of strength and I feel it more and more every day! * I am free to be strong * As a woman, I can feel strong and remain connected to my tenderness too * My heart is strong * My pelvis is strong * My bones are strong * My love is strong and my tears are strong * Now I can feel strong all the time and be feminine and flowing too * I can see that I am a soul incarnate here on Earth to feel as strong as Earth * I reclaim this flowing and weighted strength in me *now!* * Every cell in my body radiates strength * I am woman! * I am strong! * I am feminine *

I can see that I am a soul incarnate here on Earth to feel as strong as Earth * I reclaim this flowing and weighted strength in me now! * Every cell in my body radiates strength * I am woman! * I am strong! * I am feminine *...

..."She is as old and wise as the hills." The deeper feminine power of wisdom is different to the masculine power of the sharp and clear intellect. Wisdom is not information for information's sake like the intellect can be.

Chapter 4
Wisdom

Wisdom

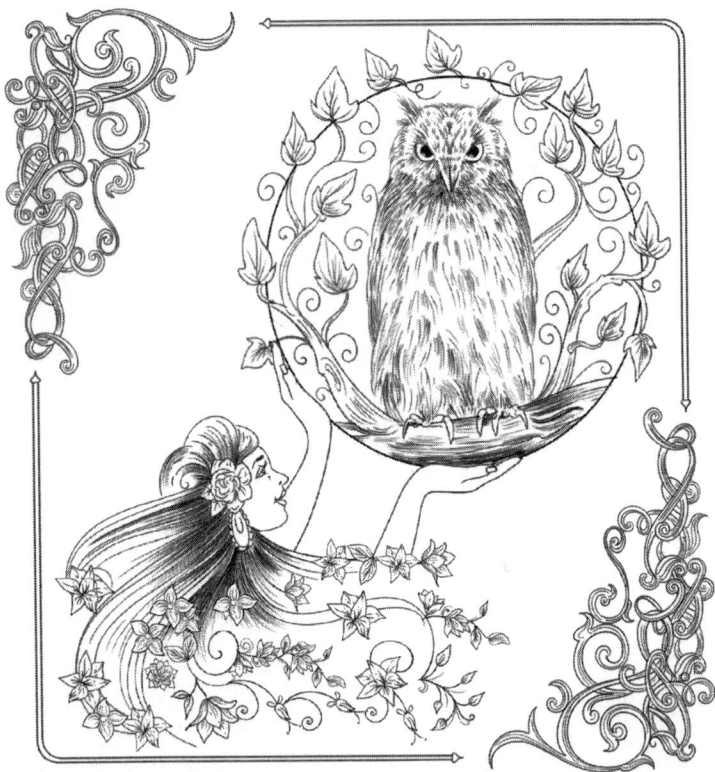

The deeper feminine power of wisdom is different to the masculine power of the sharp and clear intellect. Wisdom is not information for information's sake like the intellect can be. Wisdom is information that deeply serves humanity in some way and women are particularly endowed with quick access to the deepest *wisdom*.

Men of course have access to this too, indeed there are probably more references in various writings to the archetypal "wise old man" than there are to the "wise woman". While this is probably because the powers that be turned her into a witch, I also believe that this is because men have a propensity to find meditation and prayerful silence much easier to achieve than women (not always). I find women's minds are usually so creative that trying to stop our thoughts is like trying to stop a train with an offering of flowers. But there is a depth to the feminine that means women tend to hold the keys to wise knowing, indeed, she can be "as old and wise as the hills".

Wisdom Sees More

Men tend to be impressed by our ability to see things that they sometimes miss – whether it's finding the butter in the fridge or noticing how the great idea they are having might need to include such and such. Much of Earth is buried under the surface and thus hidden from view and who knows what treasures and troubles it holds? We women, as manifestation of the feminine principle, find it easier to access what is hidden. We just see it or feel it; or will, soon enough. We may raise our eyes to the ceiling when our man cannot see "what is obvious" but his special gift is to focus straight ahead – and get to the goal. Such is the gift of the fire element.

Men, resonating more with the Sun, have this fabulous *focusing*, straight-ahead vision and this inner drive forward, meaning they can miss what is happening on their periphery. Yes, there is another side to the Sun but there is no point looking there as it's doing the same as this side. As such, men have a tendency to see the obvious and can get caught there. It's simply not possible to focus straight ahead *and* have peripheral vision. Try it and see!

This is what we see in all successful relationships, whether business or romantic, same sex or opposite sex; the masculine in one partner has incredible focus and drive and can miss things that are not in its line of vision; the feminine in the other partner assists here with more creative peripheral vision.

Respectful Observation Is Wise

Important here for women regarding men – especially women who are particularly wise and empowered – is to observe how men do not tend to give out wisdom unless they are asked. Indeed, for a man to do this to another man would be a mark of disrespect. Women are different. We always make "helpful suggestions" to one another and we like this about each other. We chat to each other all the time and share suggestions and we love it. But men do not do this and don't like it. If we want to get on better with men, then it helps to master "respectful observation" for this is the way of the masculine.

I was listening to a comedian the other day, he was talking about men and how they are drawn to hang around each other when they are doing a task. They make a single acknowledgement to the tasker like, "Changing the tyre there?" or "New roof for this one then?" and the tasker affirms. Then the observing man stands... like the Sun... silent and shining... giving encouraging energy to the tasker. This is what the Sun does. Wisdom is when we learn to do this as women.

Getting Comfortable with Not Talking

I can hear my man laughing as I type this, as this is my weakness. But if we want to get on better with men then we have to learn to be more comfortable with silences. If we don't want silence then this is fine. We just go and mix with women friends and gabble to our hearts' content. In the polarity relationship though, we ironically disempower ourselves as women when we offer him our helpful suggestions – as our real power in this regard lies, of course, in *influencing*.

On Becoming More Wise

This is a lesson that has been so very difficult for me to learn and it's an ongoing process; to contain myself, to ground, to "Be" Earth. Here I learn to be present. To *pause* and *observe* my emotional responses and reactions and not plough in with "wisdom" and "a better way of doing things". My man is often moved and influenced by what I have to say – when I say it at the right moment. Some may raise eyes to the ceiling here with regard to male sensitivities but it works both ways. We want our man to take our femininity into account. We want them to treat us a certain way, touch us a certain way and never speak to us in this certain way or whatever. Both polarities have their sensitivities that the other must learn to value and respect if we are to live together in harmony. I speak more about this in the Feminine Power of Communication.

The Feminine Remembers

Earth itself is literally FULL of information that is here for humanity to glean for its own development and evolution. She is a veritable library. Unlike the Sun that burns stuff up and leaves no trace, Earth, being so receptive, takes stuff in and stores and holds... and remembers. How many times have we heard men complain about how we women remember everything? How many times have we heard women complain that their men don't remember? The tip here is to accept that the masculine principle does not remember – it burns information up and moves on. It's the *feminine* that remembers. Men of course have a spark of the feminine within them...

Reminding Supports the Masculine

Mark Gungor, the American comedian and motivational speaker, has taken his comedy show for married couples throughout the USA. While his and my views on spirituality differ in many ways, I deeply respect what this man knows about polarity in romantic relationships. He speaks about how **happy couples remind each other and don't mind being reminded**. And yes, it's usually (not always) the women doing the reminding; and that is okay as remembering is one of our powers. It doesn't mean we are behaving as his mother. Males, whether teenage males or adult males do need the help of the feminine to remind them as we are the ones with a decent memory and not the guys. If you are the mother of a son – especially a teenage son with his testosterone kicking in – then you'll need to remind him loads more and also remind him that he is not stupid if he needs reminding – he is turning into a man – so more focusing will be happening and less remembering what he can't see. Fire remembers nothing. It's not meant to.

Water and Earth Remember Everything

We women have no idea how powerful we are with our remembering, but men are under no illusion as to how powerful we are in this regard. The Wise Oak tree is an archetype we are all familiar with; the tree has stood there for so many hundreds of years and it has witnessed, seen and experienced so much. When you stand near an old oak tree or an ancient yew tree you can maybe sense into all that it has seen... all that it knows...

As women we are all this... And if we feel disconnected from this information, from this wisdom, then we can find other women to show us. If we affiliate ourselves with any wise women, this can mirror and awaken our own wisdom.

In the field of trauma work we also see clearly how the body remembers, on a cellular level. Nature stores the emotional and physical energy of an overwhelming event in the body and nervous system until the psyche feels safe enough to attend to it.

Menses and Menopause

That women can be so receptive and wise due to our inbuilt resonance with Gaia is a powerful place to be. Women's wisdom was recognised millennia ago when the menstruating women of the moon lodges were very much revered for their ability to have a better connection to the other dimensions during this phase of their cycle. The information gleaned was then fed back to the elders of the community to be used in leading the tribe well.

Women never lost this ability. We might not use this ability or even be aware of it but it's there. Women tend to get more powerful in this regard as they age too, with post-menopause opening us up more fully to information with a deeper connection to wisdom that has been gleaned from all levels of life.

Animal Wisdom

All the creatures on Earth correspond to the feminine principle. All animals, birds and insects have their own wisdom in the form of their "medicine". According to Native American tradition, all creatures bring their particular energy to show us that we need that *particular quality* in our lives in that moment. Like a super-intelligent feedback mechanism. The tiny and mighty ant speaks of patience and determination; the friendly and willing dog speaks of service and loyalty; the magnificent and beautiful butterfly speaks of the final stage in the process of transformation. Wiser is the woman who observes nature and takes on board the wisdom being shown.

Once, many years ago, I was treating my man a certain way. I was caught in an old pattern. Suddenly my eyes caught sight of a grasshopper on the inside of the window. Now this might not be so odd if it wasn't for the fact that I couldn't actually think where the nearest patch of grass was. So where had it come from? I lived in the middle of Cambridge UK, tarmac, concrete and buildings everywhere, no grass around, and I was indoors too! But there it was, right in front of my eyes at the very moment I was stuck in a pattern. I knew immediately what the medicine was. For grasshoppers can't hop any other way but forward. I was definitely *not* hopping forwards with my behaviour! So I paused... and chose to hop forwards and quickly updated my behaviour.

Intuitive Wisdom and Instinct

Here I make a quick and important distinction between *intuition* and *instinct*. I was shown the difference so very precisely by my Tantra teacher and I pass it on to you as I have found it to be true and helpful. I was taught that intuition stems from the throat area – where the ether or Vishuddha chakra lies. Here people will often place their hand or wave it about in this area when they speak from an intuitive place.

This is quite different from instinct, which is a lower vibration and more related to the lower chakras and instinctual knee-jerk survival *reactions*. Instinct is more about survival and so reacts quickly to the world around it like a father grabbing his child from the road away from a car. No time for thinking, just boom! Action!

To contact intuition, we need to pause... and sense inwards...

Unlike the intellect, both intuition and instinct are *bodily* experiences. Women tend to find it easier to tap into intuition as we tend to find it easier to be in our bodies. Men tend to be more instinctual due to their innately fiery and protective nature. The latter can get in the way of the former! This is a reason why men can sometimes be a liability in the birthing environment – because men tend to act instinctively to rescue which can have disastrous consequences, breaking the delicate bond between mother and baby. For a woman to birth safely, she needs a deeply wise midwife who knows how to wait and observe and follow her intuition. Even if emergency procedures are necessary, the wise midwife is best in charge.

Sometimes, when I'm working with clients, they might ask me a particular question like, "Why do I keep experiencing this?" or "Why has this not resolved yet?" Here, I get them to ask the question again but to their own intuition in their own throat area. I ask them to then pause and wait for the answer to come from within. It always does.

No Wisdom in the Head

This is different to listening to the head. When we ask the head a question we invariably ask the super ego which involves the inner critic, the judge, the persuader and the manipulator – all protector parts that link in with the reactive instinct. We don't really get wisdom from the head. But when we ask lower – to the body, to the throat or heart area – and wait there... it's wonderful what pearls rise up to the surface!

Masculine and Feminine Together See Everything

Intellectualisation can be as fresh and bright as the stars and can bring illumination to some issues for sure. Women can sometimes get caught in deep waters or stuck in the mud of an issue, and the masculine power of intellectual clarity can feel like such a relief, maybe shining light on the obvious that we hadn't been able to see due to being caught in the mire. This is another way that men and women make great partners – each offering and reflecting to the other what they themselves have more immediate access to.

In this culture there is an agenda promoting intellectualisation. It feels sterile and cold and can be dangerous as it's not connected to the heart. The fact is that *anything*, any behaviour – no matter how inhuman – can be intellectualised and rationalised. But to be a fully potentialized human being, we have to connect with the wisdom *in the body* and connect with each other in the same way.

Some Wisdom Tips

- When you find yourself in a challenging situation where wisdom is needed, "pausing" for a moment enables us to access deeper wisdom that could be vital. In a group situation (more than two people) where there is some kind of emergency that sets everyone off into a "flurry", suggesting a pause is wise indeed, enabling us to really check what needs to happen without letting reactive instinct take over. We tend to have to wait for wisdom, yes, but it's not necessarily a long wait – it might only be 5 seconds. But the breath taken in that 5 seconds enables wisdom to arrive.
- Pausing, breathing... and then grounding.... And feeling Mother Earth's energy underneath you giving you counter-pressure to your body weight, will prime you for receiving the wisdom you need.
- Making time to meditate and listen makes space for wisdom. Journaling too.

- Sleeping on a question is helpful, as overnight our soul gets information that it doesn't during the day. Contrary to what we have been told about disagreements in romantic relationships, it can often be wise to "sleep on an argument". This way, on a subconscious level we take stock of what happened and can often see more easily what we really needed or what our spouse or partner might have really needed. Wisdom takes time to appear.
- Wisdom can appear from within us or from outside of us in the form of a "message" of some sort. We might suddenly see something we haven't seen before. Or someone might text or phone, or Mother Earth may send a creature... Or from within, we might remember a dream or get a "strange" image appear in our mind. Wisdom takes many forms!

Wisdom Prayer and Affirmation

You can adjust how you do this prayer and affirmation according to how much fire you need. (See Joy Prayer and Affirmation for more information.) * Thank you for bestowing me with the wondrous gift of wisdom! * I am a very wise woman and I forgive myself for believing otherwise * The power of wisdom is so strong in me! * I feel wise in my body and wise in my soul * I fully allow myself the space and time to access this deep wisdom * More and more I gain confidence in owning the wisdom that I have within me * More and more I gain confidence in sharing the wisdom that I have direct access to * I am a soul incarnate here on earth in order to grow wiser each and every day * I reclaim this wise power in me now! * I am now reconnected to the deepest wisdom that is mine to access whenever I choose! *

I am a soul incarnate here on earth in order to grow wiser each and every day * I reclaim this wise power in me now! * I am now reconnected to the deepest wisdom that is mine to access whenever I choose! *...

...Oh my goodness! Women are creative in myriad ways but nothing can compare to the potential creativity of our own bodies.

Chapter 5
Creativity

Creativity

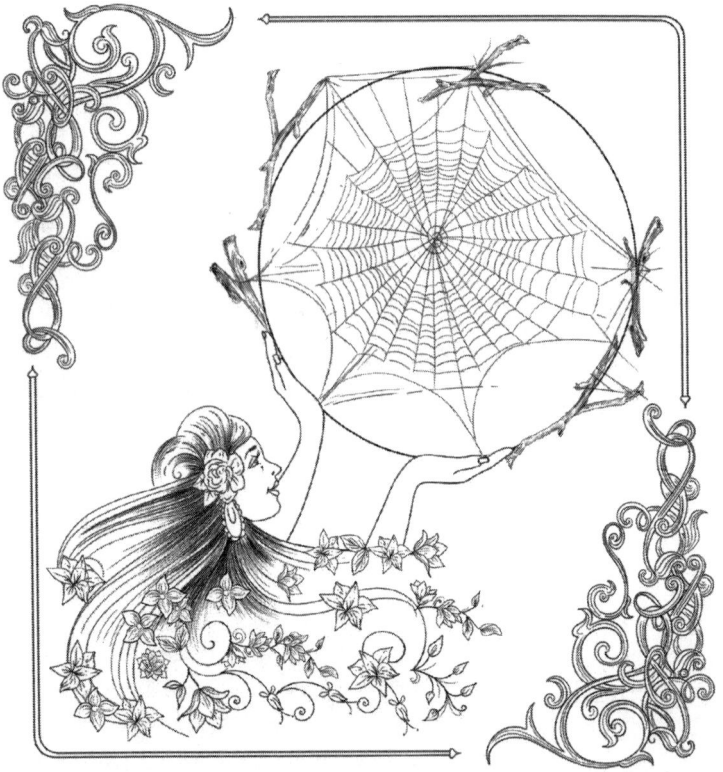

*O*h my goodness! Women are creative in myriad ways but nothing can compare to the potential creativity of our own bodies. Even if a woman has fertility issues, the *creative potential* is still there within the female body. The innate creative potential is an endowment that women receive at their incarnation, whether she goes on to co-create a baby person or not. This is really important to understand.

The Earth Creates Constantly

The feminine naturally creates stuff. She *produces* stuff. All. The. Time. She just can't help it. We see this in Nature. She is always creating and producing! She never stops creating creatures, snowflakes, new leaves, ores and minerals, fruits and vegetables and seeds and flowers and the opposite pole of bacteria, poisons and toxins. She keeps on creating a never-ending array of things animal, vegetable and mineral. And she does it all at the same time, all over Earth and all at once.

Sacred Creativity

Women don't tend to value their inherent creative abilities. Men tend to be captivated by our creativity but we seem to be unaware of the power of it. As I see it, we have been going through a phase where we have been seeing our humble every day creations as somehow of less value than paid out-in-the-world work. The drive to be accepted in the workplace has meant that women's daily creative work is no longer given value – mainly by themselves. It's even mocked as an example of pre-feminist enslavement with women laughing the loudest rather than a *divine expression of the feminine principle. Anything* that anybody makes is a Divine expression of the feminine principle. It's *all* sacred.

109

More than 100 years ago, a woman would sew, embroider, knit, crochet, make exquisite lace, and make her and her children's clothes... her ability to create beauty was as unmatched by the masculine as was his captivation of it. But we were trapped in that – by both men and other women. We were not allowed the freedom to choose and neither were men and nothing is worse than that. But now we have a different problem. We are now so busy working out in the world and then using screens to entertain ourselves that when we do "come home" to ourselves we no longer make time for our creativity. Our houses are nested with things that machines have made. We have swapped our creativity for consumption.

A Mother's Divine Creativity

When a mother makes things with her bare hands for her family, whether it is a meal or a toy for her baby or a cloth for the table – these can be holy acts. When she makes something for her baby, and she makes it with the reverence it deserves, her baby feels that on some level and a new energy is in the maternal line. When she fashions a rabbit out of a muslin square and hands it to her tearful or curious child, her child is shown the magic of the world; the magic of the feminine and the Glory of the Goddess. That child then feels in their inner being how creative and resourceful the feminine is. The infant does not notice if the stitches are uneven or if the ears do not match. That child, especially if female, gets to see how awesome *her* potential is and if that child is a boy, he gets his own experience of awe and wonder of the feminine.

So, if you have babies and children, consider making things for them. Let the stitches be wonky and let the cloth be cut unevenly as you hone your creative power.

Our Heart Is In the Creation

When a child is given a toy made by their mother – they are given a piece of her heart. And it's not too late. It's never too late. If you never made anything for your child and your child is 45 years old then you can make it now and present it to them and you can say why you made it now. And you can even say that you are sorry it's late. Not to shame yourself, but just because you might indeed feel some sorrow that you didn't feel safe enough to explore your creative power until now.

Few of us have been shown how to really know the power of our creativity and how this profoundly touches our children. It's okay to feel sad about that. It's okay to let the tears fall while you make something. Mine are falling as I write this. It is part of our power as a woman – our depth of feeling – it's the power of healing. We don't wallow in the sadness though... we allow the tears fall, and this is healing.

If you have a child, of any age, see if you can make them a little simple thing. Be humble. Be vulnerable about it. If they can't receive it, there will be a very important reason why. But at least you have become more of yourself as a woman in the creating of it. They might receive it in time...

Cake!

There is nothing like a cake that has been hand-made by a woman. I'm not saying that men cannot bake good cakes for I know they can, as I am an expert on eating cake. I am talking about the power of the feminine and how we women are especially endowed with that nurturing energy that gives a special feel to anything that we create. Especially cake. The energy of feminine nurturing and nourishment is the special ingredient that gets mixed in with all cooking by any incarnation of the feminine principle!

While my sister was doing her body psychotherapy training, she always made the same cake for her fellow students: chocolate brownie. She always made it the same way, by hand in her kitchen, and always used exactly the same ingredients from the same shop. But for one particular training module she had made it differently. She wasn't at home but was at her daughter's house. My niece was in the early stages of labour. The atmosphere was one of quiet excitement, gentle empowerment and nurturing support. Baby was born with no complications and two days later my sister was with her colleagues on her training. When her fellow students tucked into that cake, they were all enraptured. It tasted way better than usual! Markedly so. She was baffled. And then everyone else was baffled. It was mysterious. Same cake she always took. Same recipe she had used for 30 years. Same ingredients purchased in exactly the same way. No one could understand it. In the end they all agreed that some special sort of energy seemed to have been absorbed into the cake as my sister was making it and that this had somehow amplified its taste of goodness. It's not possible to research this as "quiet excitement, gentle empowerment and nurturing support" can't be patented, so no one would pay for the research!

Creativity and Highest Good

As women, we can check if our creations are in alignment with highest good. Is what we would like to create in alignment with the health of Earth and of humanity? Is what we are creating connecting us more to Earth and with the Divine, or is it causing us to *disconnect* from Earth and the Divine?

Just because we can create something specific, does it mean we should? As incarnations of the feminine principle, women are particularly gifted with broader vision here. Tending to be more embodied and less prone to intellectualisation, with more connection to feelings, gut reactions and intuition, women are oftentimes more able to sense if something is "off" or not "right". Women are less likely to rationalise a bad idea.

Men, as incarnations of the masculine principle, are so fiery that they can get very carried away with their creations; their horsepower can run away with them. Their power of motivation and focus can mean they may be more likely to miss the consequences and implications of their finished creation.

Influencing Masculine Industry

There is a very powerful energy in being male! His fiery power enables a level of focus that few women get a taste of unless they have their inner masculine high on the scale. In forgetting the coolness of the feminine, men, and indeed women, can get caught in the heat of the action and push ahead without checking if the creation is actually serving humanity.

There is so often a "cost" with many creations and the cost is often the feminine. Over-use of plastic in both products and packaging is one example; fireworks with bangers another; Teflon coated or aluminium cookware – all good ideas in part but with terrible consequences. Women can influence here more than they realise.

Let's influence our sons and lovers by expressing our joy for their innate fire. Let us express our joy and appreciation every time we see him use his fire to create something that helps others in a way that is in alignment with the Divine. I have always told my son that his fire and his creativity is a fantastic power and that I want him to use it to make things that serve his soul and help humanity.

Creating Only Beauty

On a different but connected level, we have seen creativity being both absent and misused in UK schools where we have "junk modelling" – using peoples' rubbish just for the sake of "making something". I always find this heart-breaking. How is this helping boys and girls to feel the full delights of their creativity? As humans we are amazing. We are incredibly beautiful beings and we are all here for a purpose. We all have a specific soul-task and life-purpose and as such – just like us – I think all creations that we make need to be beautiful or purposeful or ideally, both. This then reflects our inherent beauty and purpose back to us as we view or use the item. Rudolf Steiner taught that children and teenagers need the beauty of the human spirit reflected back to them constantly with whatever they create. They need help and support to create beauty. May they never make anything ugly, for the human spirit is not ugly – it is beautiful.

Creating to Heal

Conversely, it can be healing for us to work with creativity in a therapeutic way by creating a drawing, image or item that represents or depicts that which might be haunting or bothering us. Here, the thing may be very ugly indeed. I remember seeing a picture in a charity shop that was so strange that someone was mocking it. As a therapist, I could see that it was not wishful thinking on the part of the creator but perhaps an overwhelming memory that they were wanting to come to terms with.

Creating Enables Even More Creativity

So, what do you create? How do you create? What are the fruits of your labour? You might be pregnant right now with a project or idea. You might create things online or maybe you cook, knit, sew, weave or paint. Maybe you make baked goods or make jewellery for your own delight or for others, or write books! Maybe none of these things yet. But I know one thing, the more you play with creating, the more you experiment with it, the more you become connected with your power as a woman. For you are a manifestation of the feminine principle! You have so much creativity in your being! Get creating.

Symbolism of Creativity – Spider

According to the Native American tradition, the spider symbolises creativity with her constant spinning of the web – the most incredible creation! If her web gets broken she simply starts again... round and round she goes, her creation spiralling out into the world. When a spider appears in our present moment, this can be a message about our creativity. It might be that we need to hurry up and get creating, or conversely, it can be a warning that we are over-focused on a particular creation and so missing opportunities in other areas of our life. I talk more about animal wisdom in the Wisdom chapter.

Creativity and Shame

The protective super ego can keep us well away from exploring our creativity. In a bid to stop us from feeling ashamed it will have us avoid certain creative pursuits. The voice in the head can be a distraction technique that wants to stop us from getting started or it might be a constant evaluation and critiquing of our creations. Either way, it stamps on the delicate creative urge. It might tell us we don't have time. It might have us reaching for social media. It doesn't want us hurt again like when we were little or were at school.

Reclaiming Our Creativity

Here's the thing – *nothing* is as personal as the moves we make towards creating something. Whether it's clay that we mould or cloth that we sew or paper that we fold... It's all sacred... it's us being The Creator. It's also how many of us got hurt. Exploring our creativity can be a very transformative process if we aim to process the fear and shame rather than avoid it. If you feel shame about what you create or about how "good" you are at creating you might want to explore this. Is someone external to you shaming you or is it an internal voice of the super ego that is continuing the shame from the past? Where do you feel the fear and shame in your body?

Our survival instincts have us avoiding the reclamation of our creative nature. Therefore the inner fiery masculine principle must be determined and express to our super ego, "Don't worry, we are going to experiment with our creativity and no one is here to hurt us now." Go explore, play and experiment with a compassionate heart to yourself. Let the tears flow as you make and create.

Processing Old Shame To Free Creativity

By taking courage and sensing in our body where we have been holding shame, means we can focus our attention there and help it to transform. Shame is often felt in the stomach as a warm, queasy feeling, and then the face may flush with an uncomfortable warmth. There might be an accompanying sense of "pulling in and down" as if to hide. The genitals too may be holding shame around creativity because if we at some point created something that was somehow experienced as "wrong" in some way, this can actually be experienced as our very self being wrong in some way. As if our very essence is somehow wrong too. Sensing into the pelvic bowl to bring more support while we process the shame – and wherever it has been hiding – can enable it to integrate. As the shame is digested with the help of our loving awareness, your belly may even rumble as the energy is freed-up there or you might feel a "flash" of heat somewhere as your fire elements literally "burns up" the old energy. Keep sensing your pelvic bowl for support.

Using our creativity to heal ourselves is really important. Here, the things we create might feel intensely personal and not necessarily for anyone else's eyes. After a while we might share with those we trust.

How Our Creations Help Others

What if we are already creating easily and enjoy creating for others? Here an important question to ask might be, "What message am I giving?" or, "Do my creations uplift or make misery?" There is some pretty dark stuff out there for sale that has the effect of lowering our vibration that's for sure. It's good to check that we are not caught up in some indulgence of some kind. Are other people actually benefiting in a very real way when they see or view or hear or read our work? Do our creations simply affirm that we exist? Or does our work open hearts, raise vibrations and inspire and enable others? When we check our creativity this way, we begin to access the full power of the feminine!

Holding the Light

Writing this I'm thinking of Halloween. I do enjoy Halloween. I influence the atmosphere by hanging paper lanterns with real candles on my little tree to remind everybody of the light we can choose to carry into any darkness. My pumpkin becomes a pumpkin home for a gnome that was hand-made by a friend, and I made the other little pieces in his little home. I like to influence my neighbourhood in this way – showing the children a little fairyland magic and showing the mothers that they too can create this simple beauty that makes the heart sing. The children and the inner children of the adults are always utterly delighted; and then so am I.

Master the Screen Time

I thank my parents for not being able to afford a television when I was a child. I know that this has directly enabled my ability to be a super-creative being. Even now I do not own a television. I do own a laptop which I must say definitely impedes my creativity in equal amounts as enabling it as far as this book is concerned. But I thoroughly recommend keeping children away from all screens until the seventh year and even for longer if you can. Be strong with yourself and with your kids if you have them! These are tricky times to live in and parent in!

Screen anaesthesia

It helps to teach our children to notice how they feel when they are on a screen and then notice how they feel when they are not on a screen (notice how it is for yourself and then you will be able to teach your children more effectively). Get them to notice how much time they need off a screen in order to re-connect to their creativity. Try having a discussion about it. If we limit our parenting to just telling them, "Right! Get off the screen now!" this doesn't empower them to manage their own energy system and their creativity when they are away from us. (It also shocks them a bit which merely confirms to them that the anaesthetic of screen time is better, as "real life" hurts.) But, how about "Come on now, find something physically creative to do so that you can keep in touch with how amazing your creativity is." Here they can feel how you are "on their side" and wanting to "bring them up properly" which they want! And when they show you what they have created, encourage them to sense in their body how that really feels – in their own body – the difference within them between real human creativity and on-screen time. This can help them to know their energy system more deeply so that they are master of the screen and not a slave to it. Holding the boundary too does take confidence and determination. Patience coupled with support is needed to allow the child to get bored and then find their *own way* out of the post-screen haze and into empowered creative human expression. It does take time – their whole childhood! But they will thank you for it later in life.

Our innate creativity as women is powerfully influential.

Some Creativity Tips

- If you are already actively creative, you might want to notice how it feels in your body that you are like this. How does it feel that you can use this power? It helps to really *know* the experience of yourself as a creative woman. So, you might notice a subtle or even powerful sensation in your heart or even your womb. Or maybe your belly in general.
- If you are creating to heal yourself, it might help to know and feel in your body how it is helping you, to really sense how it's enabling you. Feel what is opening up in your body. Sensing into the physical sensation of this...
- If creating for others, you might want to check that what you are doing delights you as much as it serves others. Keep your vibe high. Create in a way that raises the vibration of those that see your work. Create to help humanity raise its vibe!
- You might want to experiment whilst being in a meditative

state of peace and calm. From here you might want to see if you can share that vibe beyond the walls of the room you are in – literally imagine your loving vibe extending out to uplift others too.

- If you are new to being creative, consider making gifts for people you love and who love you, at first. Starting with those you feel safest with, to get you used to this power being seen by others.

Creativity Prayer and Affirmation

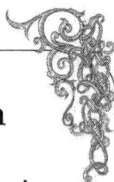

You can adjust how you do this prayer and affirmation according to how much fire you want to create within yourself (see Joy Prayer and Affirmation). * Thank you for bestowing in me the wondrous power of creativity! * I am a creative being and I forgive myself for believing otherwise! * The power of my creativity is so strong in me * I am free to be creative! * I begin to embrace my creativity in all its forms! * I can see that I am a soul incarnate here on earth for a rich and creative experience! * I am free to create! * I reclaim this *flowing* power in me now and I feel this deeply in my body! * I am now reconnected to bountiful creative energy! Yes. Yes. Yes! * I create to heal myself * I create to heal myself and others * My creations influence the world and make the world a better place *

I am now reconnected to bountiful creative energy! Yes. Yes. Yes! * I create to heal myself * I create to heal myself and others * My creations influence the world and make the world a better place*...

...A new word for this chapter: empleasured. Every woman has been endowed with the power of pleasure and can indeed live an empleasured life. Everything about us is made for experiencing pleasure. We women are stacked with pleasure-making potential for us to choose to amplify according to our desires.

Chapter 6
Pleasure

Pleasure

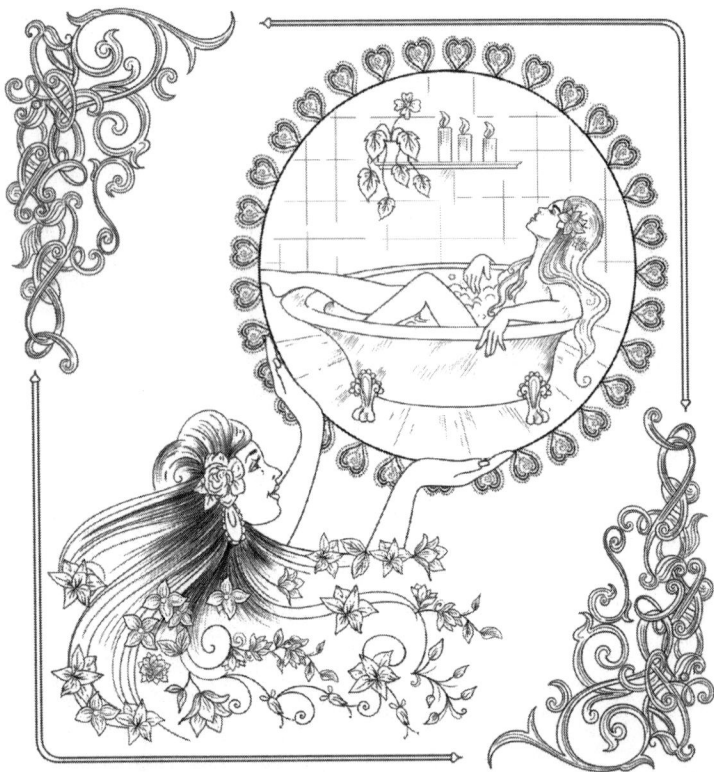

A new word for this chapter: empleasured. Every woman has been endowed with the power of pleasure and can indeed live an empleasured life. Everything about us is made for experiencing pleasure. We women are stacked with pleasure-making potential for us to choose to amplify according to our desires.

As little girls, most of us were not shown our feminine capacity for pleasure and our mothers and grandmothers maybe did not know it either. We were perhaps shown a mundane life. Even in a "happy childhood", if we were not shown the pleasures that our little body was capable of then I say we were shown a mundane life. Many of us were brought up to have our pleasure dial turned down.

Women's Bodies Are Made for Pleasure

Here's the thing. As women we *are* pleasure. We are made for pleasure every day. Our very anatomy is even made for pleasure! I'm not just talking of the amazing clitoris with its 15,000 nerve endings, but our *whole body* and psyche is made for feeling pleasure. Our skin is even made for pleasure. Did you know that it is actually thinner than men's skin? Funny how we haven't been told this, huh? That our skin is much more sensitive to touch and caressing. Yup! Everything tends to feel much more pleasurable to us women. Yes, he feels pleasure too for sure, but he is more set up to be *giving* pleasure and so this works well, as men are wired for service and love to see their woman in a state of pleasure that they are responsible for, as this makes them feel really potent and powerful! Men's skin being a bit thicker is also perfect considering one of the main powers of the masculine is "protection", and so if men's skin was as sensitive as ours, he wouldn't be so powerful in this regard.

Women Feel *More*

Due to our receptivity, women tend to feel things more deeply; the feel of our favourite beauty products on our skin, the feel of the warm grass under our naked feet, the cat brushing past our bare legs. All very sensual... and can feel utterly amazing to us. Put a guy in the same situation and he'll like it for sure, but we tend to like it more! Some men even find a lighter touch too "tickly". But to us women – especially if we are truly present and sensing into our body – it might feel sweetly erotic. If we allow ourselves to sink deeply into any of the aforementioned pleasures – and turn the pleasure dial up one or two notches at a time, life really becomes even more pleasurable.

Sensual and Tactile

Women tend to be more sensual and tactile. You can see us when we are shopping, as we always stroke and handle the things we are interested in and attracted to. "Ooo I love this!" we say, as we pick something up or stroke it with our hands. Or we visit a friend's house and we admire her new throw on her sofa with our hands in a sensual way. Or we feel and stroke the garment that we are knitting as we create it. Men don't tend to do this. They don't tend to stroke the wheel as they change it or stroke the jumpers in the shop as they consider a purchase. It tends to be much more about achieving a goal; yes, I like this jumper. Take it to the till to pay. Job done.

Including Our Yoni in Our Pleasure

Our whole life can be a pleasure-filled experience. Many of us don't tend to include our yoni in our everyday moments. Many of us have been shown to only bring awareness to this area when we make love. The trouble with this disconnection is that it minimises our pleasure and also affects lovemaking as it restricts blood flow each day.

Earth and Water Chakras

I use this term "Yoni" here as it includes the whole area – vulva and vagina. The yoni also includes the feminine chakras – the earth and water chakras; otherwise known as the first and second chakras. These chakras are important energy centres. Information about these energy centres has been hidden from us for millennia and thus the importance and relevance that these centres bring to our health and our life have also been hidden and denied. There are different models that locate the chakras in different places. For example, some models locate the earth chakra at the tip of the tail bone and the water chakra at the base of the sacrum. I use the Tantric model, as this is where I personally feel them; the earth or first chakra is experienced in the perineum, between the vagina and anus and the water chakra is experienced just above the clitoris.

When we choose to become more aware of our yoni on a daily basis, this brings more pleasure into our life. We feel more whole. The process of love-making, then, is not so far away from our everyday existence because we are generally more alive and living in our sexuality.

Feminine Sexuality

By the term "sexuality" I mean how it is to be in the fulness of our feminine sex. When a woman is embodied into her whole being and everywhere is included, her yoni, her breasts, her ankles, her neck, her belly... this is her full connection to her sexuality; how she embraces her feminine body.

Layers of Pleasure

The pleasure-filled sensations of femininity can feel like anything from a tidal wave whooshing through us up to the most sublime and exquisite sensations. Women have the potential to experience varying degrees of pleasure throughout the body, and this naturally *includes* the yoni.

There are reasons why we may not feel comfortable with this. We may unconsciously deaden ourselves. This kind of pleasure, this deep libidinal force, is an energy that originally needed support from our mother. Ideally, this happens as the mother simply *knows* this experience in her being and is in touch with this energy in herself as she bonds with her baby. Ideally, the mother is in touch with her own empleasured forces and so shows her baby with her very own feminine presence.

Pleasure and Politics

Of all the powers of the feminine this one can be the most challenging power as it is the one that until now has been most deeply suppressed by our familial patterning and by global politics. We are told the Suffragettes started the change in this but they themselves seemed to have had little support for becoming fully empleasured and joyful Goddesses. Emeline Pankhurst's father himself is reported to have said of her, "What a pity she was not born a lad." While this acknowledged her battle to get into the male-dominated workplace, her father had completely dismissed her Divine and most wonderful femininity. He had also ignored her deeper, perhaps unconscious pain at not being truly adored as a beautiful and creative female with her own innate, wondrous cornucopia of empleasured and joyful delights.

Our Grandmother's Pleasure Dial

As women, if our mother's or grandmother's pleasure dial was turned down low, we would have followed suit. This happens because as babies we naturally bond so totally with all that our mother thinks and feels. The energy of the female line shows us how to "be" feminine and all that this means on a deeply experiential and feeling level. This gets locked into our human energy field and our nervous system. Was it safe to be sexually alive in your family? Was it safe for your mother and your grandmother?

Our Own Pleasure Dial

Knowing the hidden entanglements of the maternal line and disentangling them can be a huge step to freeing up our own pleasure (and to freeing up other feelings too) as a woman. With our naturally risky childhood behind us, we are free to fully explore the delights of our femininity. We don't do our maternal line any favours by being asleep from the waist down. Yes, we may feel closer to our mother and our ancestors in staying entangled and we may feel loyal in doing so, but we are not free when we do this and often even crippled. Likewise, they too are held by our entangling with them, for they cannot move on in the Spirit world if we are holding their energy.

Fathers

And fathers too, in order to support their daughters' connection to her experience of full pleasure, need to have good, clear boundaries. A father needs to make sure that he doesn't attempt to get his unmet emotional needs or his sexual needs met through his daughter. In health, he would be naturally closer to his wife or his lover and get his emotional and sexual needs met through her. Unconsciously using his daughter to fulfil these needs would sexually stifle her. She needs to be given the space to find the fullness of her empleasured nature without that being used in any way whether this is done consciously or not.

To heal this kind of confusion, a woman may need to work with reclaiming her sexual energy as her own. Clearly saying "No" and using her hands to push away and feel her own sexual energy as her *own* sexual energy for her *own* pleasure first. From here, she can then choose to share this special energy only with people who will not abuse it.

Inner Masculine Can Block Pleasure

Another way a woman can become tuned out of her pleasure is when she relies too strongly on her inner masculine. If she works way too hard or does a job where she has to over-focus, then there is a cost and the cost can be her pleasure. I think it's really important for a woman not to work too hard; or if she has to work hard, to factor in a *lot* of self-care. We are made for pleasure not toil! Work soft and strong like a river flowing. Hard is testosterone and masculine principle. Our culture is very much created this way but it is not our future. At the moment, we women are still trapped really. We are either trapped at home and not appreciated by ourselves or each other as amazingly influential, creative beings, or we are trapped at work, cut off from our pleasure and creativity, relying hard on the masculine principle to contribute to huge mortgages and complex lifestyles. Ask a woman when she last felt pleasure and she may laugh and then maybe weep...

Pleasure and the Super Ego

If we were not shown how to live in pleasure when we were little, our super ego will surely have something to say about it when we try it as a woman. This can leave us feeling ashamed and uncomfortable about allowing more pleasure. The super ego is an old defence that protected us when we were little by making sure we followed the status quo. Becoming aware of the super ego and learning to deal with it can feel very empowering! We might say to it, "I know you are wanting to distract me from feeling pleasure because you are fearful of this new experience, but it's safe to feel it now."

As women it is always safe to explore our connection with pleasure. How much pleasure can we allow ourselves? Tantrics speak of it being possible for women to "make love with the world".

But Isn't This Dangerous?

Many women fear that if they fully connect to the full sweetness of themselves, they will somehow be taken advantage of by men; or that men will somehow sense this and treat them disrespectfully or pounce like a cat on a mouse. This belief might be from historical experience that needs to be attended to in order to be free, or it may come from an entanglement from the maternal line. Additionally, this kind of belief is also another big trick of the super ego as an attempt at protection. As we begin to uncover a new identity as an empleasured woman, our super ego might attempt to scupper this.

From my own experience both with myself and with clients, I have found that when we explore deeper levels of pleasure in our feminine body, this actually brings *respect* from

131

men. Sonja Maria Devi – who has worked with this energy with thousands of women, helping them awaken into the fullness of their pleasure – has also found that these fears are unfounded. I think this is a direct reflection of the depth of power of fully connected feminine sexuality – men respect it and admire it and are captivated by it. Health begets health.

Raising Our Vibe Protects Us

Keeping our pleasure dumbed down and thus our vibration low does not protect us from the darkness in this world; but raising our vibration by healing ourselves and allowing more joy and pleasure certainly helps to keep us safer due to the other natural law of "like attracts like".

Men Need Us Empleasured

In terms of ramping up our pleasure in the bedroom, men find our capacity to feel and express pleasure incredibly exciting. Men tend to feel captivated when they experience our pleasure in everyday life or in the bedroom. This is especially true if they have taken some part in enabling that, or even if they think they have enabled that. The more we are empleasured the more he feels like a king.

Men, as incarnations of the masculine principle, need to be engaged in the experience of our pleasure. This helps them to come down into their heart and out of the trap of their head. It's an organic win-win situation. All this pleasure feeling is not just a powerful thing to be experiencing. It also puts us in a powerful position as women. This must not be abused by ourselves or used to manipulate. If we use our body to manipulate then this means we have not healed the wounds of our inner child and it will break the trust our man has for us. The pleasure and innate eroticism in our body is a sacred thing that must not be used as a bargaining tool. This is the same for men's bodies too.

I've mentioned the word "erotic" here, and this word is from the Greek name "Eros" who was the God of Love. For me, this keeps the term nicely away from modern-day uses in the sex industry and keeps it way up high in the realms of the Divine, where sensual pleasure, love and eroticism are all expressions of the sacred feminine.

Taking a Slice of Pleasure Pie

We have to claim our pleasure. We have to *want* it again. It doesn't come running up the garden path one day. We have to go and *get* it. Make space for it. Sink into it, allow it. This is where we need the inner masculine to help with his determination. If you have a crazy busy life and resonate with the paragraph above, try this:

Before you leave for work in the morning, put a fresh towel or two on the bathroom radiator; choose your favourite oils and place them as a massage salon would. Arrange them so that they will greet you later. Grab anything else that delights you, like a certain crystal or ornament or something. Get those bath salts out or whatever else you could pop in your bath and totally set the room up ready for your return later. Notice how it feels in your body to do this. Then go to work and do your thing. Notice how it feels to be at work knowing that this is waiting for you at home. And as soon as you get in, run the bath and enjoy the pleasure. Don't betray yourself by not doing it or you might never do this again.

Notice the whole of this experience *in your body* as you do it.

Take Your Pleasure

If you are a woman and you have a job that requires a lot of you – sister, it is your birthright to help yourself to a nice big slice of daily pleasure pie. But you have to take it. *No one* will serve this up to you. It's not their job. It's your job. Being a woman is a big responsibility and the world needs us enlivened and full of pleasure. Don't wait for your loved ones to give this to you. No matter how much they love you it's not their job. It's part of your power as woman to make sure you put yourself first and grab that pleasure pie and scoff it down!

My Pleasure List

Some things that get me feeling the pleasure in my female body:

- Using Dr Hauschka skin products (Biodynamic and organic – yum!)
- I often check that my cat's fur is still soft. It always is. Best check again.
- I have woollen carpets
- I use (some) Marie Kondo methods in my home
- I love to shower
- I make sure I keep very warm and snug in winter; when I go out I wear merino underwear (this is – of course – on top of my pretty underwear)
- I lie in the sun naked for ½ hour in the spring and summer
- I eat one or two squares of dark chocolate a day
- I always wear comfy shoes
- I try not to work "hard". I work as soft as I can.

Exercise: Awakening Ourselves to Pleasure

• A way to start with just gently moving your hips... scoop
  upwards and tilt backwards... to gently awaken... as we might
  gently awaken a dear friend from a deep sleep if it were time to
  go do something fun together – we might rub their back and
  gently rock their shoulders if they didn't immediately respond.

• Movement is key. Dancing and flowing... leaning and
  stretching... swaying and stirring your pelvis like you might
  stir cosmic soup. The positive pole of the hips are the
  shoulders so really move them too and open up your chest
  as well. Keep moving... keep loosening... keep opening... like
  moving a knotted piece of rope so that the knot is easier to
  undo... keep moving... take a warm shower and move around
  under the water spray... the feminine is very much a moving,
  flowing, unfolding thing... become a flowing river... gently
  twisting and moving and awakening your body... you could
  try doing this for 5 minutes a day for a week and record
  your results in a Pleasure Journal. Here you could state your
  fantasies that bring you pleasure as well... how do you feel
  that pleasure in your body? Is it tingling or warm? Or cool?

The cat can perfectly exemplify pleasure. The way they lie... and
stretch... and purr... and "purr-yow" and lie in full, stretched-
out sweet-abandon in the dust or the grass or the bed or on the
floor... We can just *see* and feel that they are in their pleasure
zone and we can choose to resonate with that. The cat's *whole
body* is alive and writhing with the pleasure of existence.

How Can I Awaken to More Pleasure?

You can also ask your body "what would help to awaken you

more?", "What would support your aliveness?" Trust what it says... trust the still small voice or the image that comes up from your body. Not the loud voice in your head from the super ego that screams scary stuff at you to keep you the same. You know deep down in your being what will help you awaken more. Your body is made of nature... it knows what it needs to unwind, let go, release and wake-up.

Some Pleasure Tips

- Try slowing right down. I've noticed that the faster I move through life, the more disconnected I become. I was taught in my training that "speed is demonic".
- As I touch and stroke things, I feel the different textures and sense into my body as I do this...
- When we eat, we might want to really slow down and take our time to relish the different flavours.
- When we gaze upon any beauty – an amazing tree, the sunset, a plant, a lovely house made into a home, the amazing sky, the stars – we can try really drinking that in and noticing how this feels in our body. How does that amazing sunset feel in your body? When you look at that marvellous tree, what happens in your body? When you see a beautiful dress or beautiful fabric, what happens in your body?
- I smell everything. I'm forever stickin' my nose in a rose! I feel it in my body as I do this! We were made for smelling flowers! Essential oils are great too. Really good ones. Not synthetic ones – as I think we inherently sense not to really breathe these in too deeply – but really good oils that you know you can smell right up into your brain.

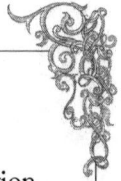

Pleasure Prayer and affirmation

You can adjust how you do this prayer and affirmation according to how much fire you want to create within yourself (see Joy Prayer and Affirmation). * Thank you for bestowing me with the wondrous gift of pleasure! * It is safe for me to begin to feel pleasure * I begin to allow it more and more! * I am indeed an empleasured being of juicy womanliness! * The power of pleasure is so delightful in my being and I allow it now! * I am willing and able to feel my body awaken to pleasure * I am a soul incarnate here on earth for a rich and pleasure-filled experience! * I am free to feel pleasure! * I reclaim this *flowing* energy in me NOW! * I am now reconnected to bounteous pleasure energy! Yes. Yes. Yes. *

I am a soul incarnate here on earth for a rich and pleasure-filled experience! * I am free to feel pleasure! * I reclaim this flowing energy in me NOW! * I am now reconnected to bounteous pleasure energy! Yes. Yes. Yes.*...

...Nature is incredibly beautiful. The Sun is of course a very handsome and magnificent fella, but "beautiful" is perhaps not how we might describe the Sun. We tend to use other adjectives.

Chapter 7
Beauty

Beauty

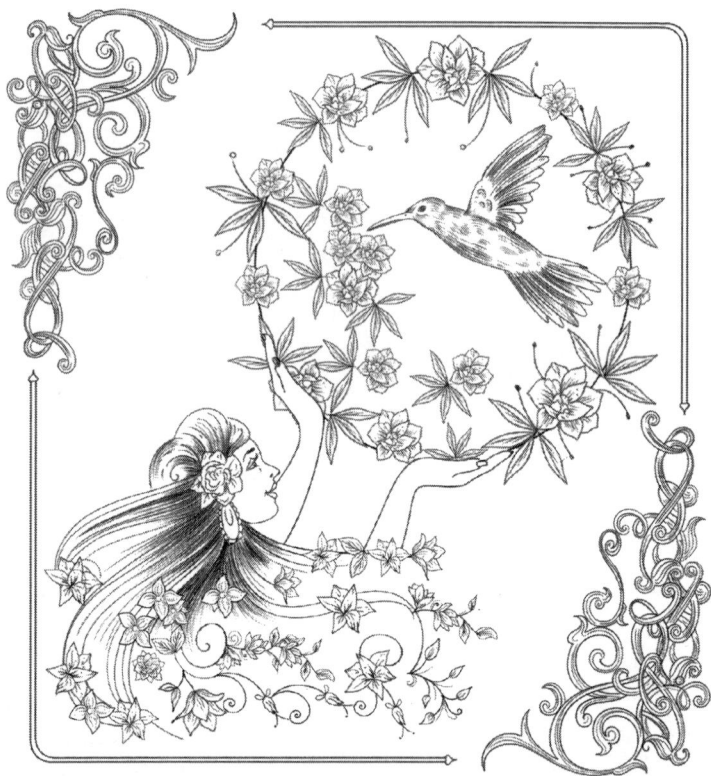

*N*ature is incredibly beautiful. The Sun is of course a very handsome and magnificent fella, but "beautiful" is perhaps *not* how we might describe the Sun. We tend to use other adjectives. But the Earth plane *is* simply beautiful... and more so on a sunny day when the awesome rays of the bright and illuminating Sun shine down onto her luscious and fertile lands and seemingly *ignite* her beauty. Such is the power of polarity!

Exquisite Beauty

In addition to her beautiful mountains, open plains and dark forests, Nature also has great intricacies. There are little exquisite bits! Teeny weeny forms that are so delicate... the tiny petals on the violet flower, the mother of pearl inside the piece of sea shell, the crystalline form of a tiny quartz...

All Women Are Beautiful

As the incarnation of the feminine principle, we women have a particular tendency to be beautiful! It was Mr Van Gogh who apparently stated that there was no such thing as an ugly woman. I find that what some may judge as "plain" or "not a model", there is still a beauty there – she just can't help it. We are generally quite good to look at – especially naked. But just as Earth has gravity, women tend to look "inwards" rather than "outwards" like the Sun, and so we tend to get lost in what we consider our "flaws". Our men are mostly baffled by this and feel powerless to help us. And they and our friends will never agree that we are less than beautiful. Some women may appear to be particularly beautiful. But all women are seen to be beautiful by their lover or partner.

Considering the sperm and the egg as examples of the two principles, we can see that the egg is, again, the fairer sex. Even a spider's egg is beautiful. Even a snail egg is beautiful; its shape, its lustre, its translucence that seems to glow. Whether perfectly spherical or more "egg shaped", the beauty is simply there and one can gaze upon it for a time and wonder at its huge potential and the cosmic intelligence lying therein.

Beauty Heals

Research now clearly shows that beautiful environments have an effect on our health and on our development as human beings. Studies have shown how the brain is positively affected and how the nervous system becomes calm around nature and beauty – around big trees especially. Mountainous regions, too, and lake-land areas all really support healthy brain functioning, enabling humanity to thrive and our spirits to lift. People find it much easier to meditate in beautiful environments too. But even the man-made can be beautiful – Venice is one of my favourite places and it is so interesting to me that even though there is barely a tree in sight, somehow there is enough man-made beauty in that place to lift the vibe anyway!

Beauty Raises Our Vibe

There is much evidence now to prove that beauty anywhere is healing. A beautiful home helps too – I am a great fan of Marie Kondo. She understands the power of beauty. She shows us that it's not just having a "beautiful house"; it's about the arrangement of things inside the home that determines the beauty. Love comes in here too. Things placed in a beautiful and conscious way is an expression of love. When things are placed in a beautiful way in a space, the soul can somehow settle more easily in the physical body. Beauty resources us and replenishes us. Our body opens and relaxes as we observe a

142

beautiful plant in an attractive pot, or when we enter a room that has been consciously and beautifully arranged, or when we see a beautiful work of art. Beauty lifts us. Beauty helps us to alchemise into a higher version of ourselves and heal.

More Stress – Less Beauty

Interestingly, when a woman is stressed, her fire element expands and she becomes more masculine and conversely less beautiful. Have you noticed this? We become less receptive and "harder". Fire ascends and water descends and we lose our lustre, our juiciness. The masculine principle and the fire element are related to *protection*. So, when women get stressed, our fire kicks in to protect us. Aren't we amazing? We don't look quite so beautiful but we do feel safer. A stressed woman cannot really relax into her feminine powers – as she is having to rely more on her masculine powers. She becomes her own knight in shining armour to take care of the show, and keep herself safe. Her real beauty will not shine through again until she lays her sword down, relaxes and lets go... into her flowing and deep waters.

And the woman whom we might not consider beautiful at all is all this when she realises that she was never _seen_ nor _held_ as beautiful. That her mother, fresh from a disempowered birth, never had her oxytocin flush that makes the whole world seem beautiful. Her mother never got the chance to hold this baby in that enraptured blissful gaze that a new mother ideally will. And her father never adored her or called her princess. And there... in this agonising realisation, her grief releases the beauty and she glows. A beauty hidden all these years in the denial of her pain at not being seen as the exquisite beauty that she was. Her tear-wet face now alive with rosy glow and her heart now opening to herself, this woman is now the most beautiful woman in the world!

Superficial Beauty

When beauty is taken in isolation – away from the many powers of the feminine – we get superficiality. We get shallow, disempowered behaviour and no sense of the *many* powers of the feminine and how this can change the world. I call it "porny" energy. Everything has been tidied up on her body and she looks like one of those rose gardens at a posh country house that you pay money to walk around and "admire", but the energy of the place can be a bit overdone and dead. There is no magic. The garden is not "alive" with the powers that you get in a wild garden where many more elements are supported.

Don't get me wrong. I enjoy my lipstick and heels – I don't go out without my lipstick on – but it is now obsessive in our culture; fake eyebrows, fake lips, fake eyelashes, fake noses, fake breasts, extreme waxing, injections of stuff taken off our thighs and injections of other stuff shoved back in to make your butt look "uppsy" – and somewhere inside she feels dead.

Natural Beauty

I remember meeting a woman I knew in a shop in town; she was with her daughter. This woman was a very natural woman herself and big into nature and natural living. Her daughter was about three and was exquisitely beautiful and I said so. The mother then "corrected" me with her need to affirm her daughter's other qualities. I totally understood where she was coming from but it was almost as if she was trying to repair the statement I had made as if what I had suggested was wrong. I came away from that interaction feeling strongly that the feminine IS beautiful and that it's *okay* to be beautiful. To try and deal with the media and the beauty industry by taking the beauty out of the feminine is impossible. Because women are so beautiful and so like Nature! There is such an inherent need for girls and women to *feel* as beautiful as Nature. It's part of feminine sexuality.

Tell Your Daughter of Her Beauty

One way we can address this with our children is by telling our daughter that she is beautiful whatever state she is in; when she wakes up in the morning all messy and blurry-eyed, or when she is hot and sweaty from playing in the garden, and even when she has a bogie. If we only tell her she is beautiful when she is "scrubbed up" then we don't help her and we don't really *see* her.

As women... as the very incarnation of the Divine feminine principle – there is simply beauty down to our very bones.

Protecting Beauty

A woman may unconsciously turn against her femininity and her beauty to protect herself. Many years ago, I knew a young woman who had unconsciously made her body look ugly. Her father had been sexually interested in her and thus her femininity was experienced as a dangerous thing. The innate intelligence of her body and psyche created lesions on her skin in an attempt to "put him off her". Staggering intelligence. This kind of thing can also be traced back down the maternal line leaving femininity and femaleness cloaked in shame and feeling like it's a treacherous thing that must be controlled, denied or, these days – even removed. Once the time is right, in the safety of a good enough healing context, a woman can find her inner knight by finding a safe place to finally find her "No" and thus her own boundaries. Here she can reclaim the delights and riches of her deepest feminine sexuality – and the depth of her beauty – for *herself*.

"I Am Beautiful"

And to dare to say that we ourselves are beautiful? Would we dare? Well, I am beautiful. There. I've said it. You do not know me. I have all sorts of areas of myself that are fabulously imperfect because I am a woman. But I am still beautiful. I'd love to start a trend – women acknowledging their beauty.

Naked Is Beautiful

Our naked body is a thing to admire. Ask any woman if she'd rather see images of a woman's naked body or a man's naked body and many will say a woman's – because our bodies are simply more beautiful to look at. Unfortunately, the porn culture (i.e. those in the industry and the consumers of it) has gone crazy now with women using their beauty in a way that is not for highest good. Yes, it is powerful to have a woman's body, it's very powerful. Men in particular have a direct relationship with the fire element which means that they have a strong relationship with the head and the eyes in particular. This means that men are more visually stimulated in a way that women aren't. (Really, we have no idea.)

Porn and Beauty

The porn industry is where the beauty of the feminine form is abused. Porn teaches girls to be hysterical and disconnect from their body, and it teaches boys to use feminine beauty to ejaculate. This is not helping anyone's development as a human being and is keeping us stuck in lower states of consciousness.

Porn teaches men to "pop one out" in reaction to the beauty of the feminine form. Cases of premature ejaculation and erectile dysfunction are now at a record high. Porn teaches women to be disconnected from their highly receptive body and psyche. This doesn't show either the gals or the guys how to master sexual energy. To be a good lover, a man actually needs to *slow down* his urges in response to the beauty he beholds and bring his woman slowly to the boil. He needs to be shown how to *rein-in* and *ground* his energy, connect to his heart, and thus *step further* into his manhood. This in turn increases the charge in the polarity and gives us women a better sexual experience which then gives him an even better experience too. It's another win-win situation. Ejaculation just stops everything.

Beauty and Real Love-Making

I have found both personally and in my work with others that the more connected a woman is to her vagina the more beautiful she feels and the more beautiful she becomes! Kim Anami and Sonja Maria Devi are both super busy helping women feel even more connected and even more beautiful. When we are even more aware of our vagina, our beauty is supercharged! When we awaken to new levels of sexual awareness, men then get the chance to "polish up" their act in order to meet their woman. Men like to be given a challenge and be given the chance to shine to please their beautiful lady. Everybody wins when women develop and awaken.

Beauty and Culture

We are all naturally attracted to beauty and to beautiful people. A woman's natural, magnetic beauty organically influences everyone around her. Without her even trying. When a woman raises the bar by developing herself further – just by her deeply connecting with her own feminine, beautiful nature – she becomes a powerful force in the world.

Some Beauty Tips

- You might like to try a simple Mantra like "I am beautiful."
- What can aid our healing around our beauty is to try the Tapping intro; "Even though part of me believes that I am not beautiful, I still love, accept and forgive myself" (said slowly and with meaning). This intro part of Tapping is done by Tapping with three fingers on the karate chop point on the side of the hand while repeating variations of the statement three times. Doing this, whilst perceiving our emotions and feelings in our body as we do this can be very healing. Alternatively, simply feeling compassion for ourselves that we may have believed that we were not beautiful – puts our brain and nervous system into a healing mode.
- When I remember, I pause when I observe beauty... and sense into my body the experience of beholding the beauty before me. It could be perceived as a meditation or even as a prayer.
- If I see a woman who is wearing something beautiful or whose hair I find beautiful, I might make the effort to verbalise this to her. I always remember walking behind a beautiful lady in town. She was a larger lady and seemed very self-assured as she walked along in her skirt suit and high heels and she had the most amazing calves and ankles! As I walked past her I took the risk and told her I thought she had amazing legs and she was utterly delighted. We were both lifted by the interaction.
- How do we receive compliments about our own beauty? What happens in your body when someone acknowledges your beauty or acknowledges your clothes or belongings as beautiful? Do you freeze? Does someone's compliment trigger a super ego attack? If so, what is your super ego frightened of here? What might you need to attend to so that you can now receive compliments and feel safe to do so?

- I have purchased some super essential oils and I keep them in my bathroom. After my shower, I choose one or maybe two oils and add one drop to the palm of my hand and then add a "shloop" of organic coconut oil. I then rub my hands together and lightly massage this onto my face and then what's left goes all over the rest of my body. I do this simple routine every morning with an intention of love, acceptance and healing and it *feels* beautiful.

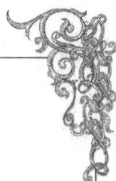

Beauty Prayer and Affirmation

You can adjust how you do this prayer and affirmation according to how much fire you need. (See Joy Prayer and Affirmation for more information.) * Thank you for bestowing me with the wonderful gift of feminine beauty! * It is safe for me to see myself as beautiful! * I allow my beauty more and more! * I am indeed a beautiful being of womanliness! * I forgive myself for believing otherwise! * Even the teeniest parts of me that are hidden are beautiful * My yoni is beautiful * My vagina is beautiful * My heart is beautiful * My body is beautiful * My mind is Beautiful * I am beautiful inside and out! * My soul is beautiful too and I am incarnate here on Earth for a rich and beautiful female experience! * My feminine spirit is beautiful * I am now free to be beautiful! * I reclaim this power of beauty *now*! * Yes! Yes! Yes! *

I am beautiful inside and out! * My soul is beautiful too and I am incarnate here on Earth for a rich and beautiful female experience! * My feminine spirit is beautiful * I am now free to be beautiful! * I reclaim this power of beauty now! * Yes! Yes! Yes!*...

...Being with each other and truly connecting with our hearts is when we use the feminine power of relationship. This, like all feminine powers, is what makes life feel really good! The feminine power of relationship is the "glue" which connects us all together.

Chapter 8
Relationship

Relationship

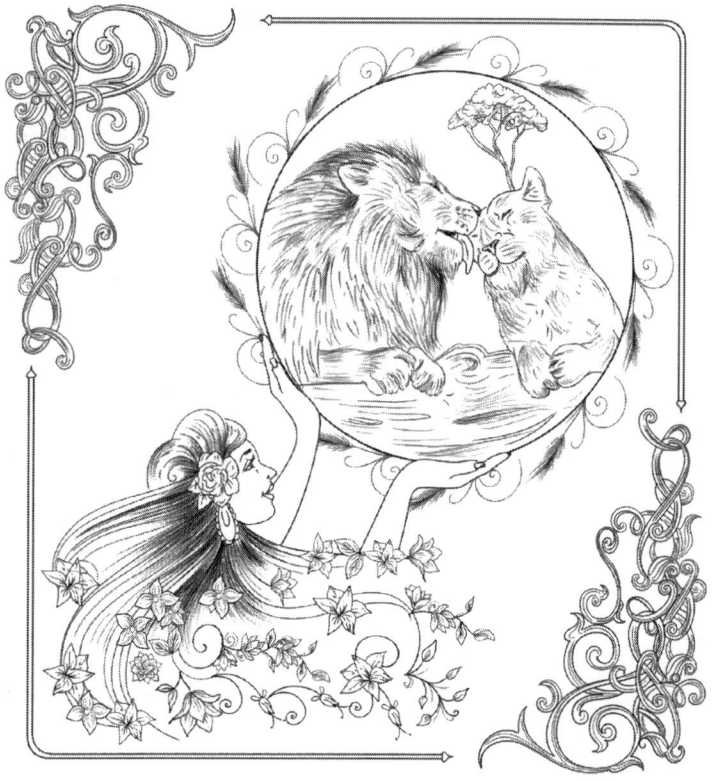

*B*eing with each other and truly connecting with our hearts is when we use the feminine power of relationship. This, like all feminine powers, is what makes life feel really good! The feminine power of relationship is the "glue" which connects us all together. We might be sitting with someone or next to someone but we are not truly in relationship with them unless we are connecting in a real way, and the feminine power of relationship is what does this. Relating seeks to know how the other *really* is. When we are using this power, we want to *hear*. We want to *share*. We want to *connect* in an honest and heart-felt way and this can feel vulnerable and tender as much as it can feel joyful.

The feminine power of relationship is never bossy and controlling as these states do not really include any acknowledgement of the feelings and the experiences of the other. Nor is relationship domineering or dismissive, and neither is it angry, for even anger hides and detracts from primary feelings of fear underneath which, if expressed, can deepen our connection with each other.

In relationship we never tell someone what to do. If we do, the other might oppose us in a glorious act of polarisation! In relationship we might express what would delight our heart and then the other might be influenced! We can do no more than state what would bring us joy!

Relating With Nature

Mother Nature is in constant relationship with herself. There is constant interaction and responsiveness. As human beings, our happiness depends on our being in relationship with Nature. Health studies galore show us the science behind our relationship with Nature and in her relationship to us. I notice how my garden appears to beam in delight and "brighten" as I attend to it; and I know if my brain was wired up to a monitor at this time it would show that my brain is as equally positively affected by my attending to my garden.

Our bodies show this as we, too, have an incredibly intelligent system of inter-relationship that happens through all the pathways, structures and hormone messengers in our body, and the bio feedback is impressive. These constant inter-relationships - whether in our body or on Earth - are mind-blowing. When we really look at it, we can see how this could only be created and organised by some Divinely Great Intelligence.

The Feminine Relates Easily

As incarnation of the feminine, we women tend to relate well. We tend to find it *easier*. Not always for sure. I know plenty of times when I've been mute or plain bitchy. But this general ability women have to be more emotionally articulate is very much a feminine way. This power in us is much admired by men young and old, and even teenage boys admire their female peers for their ability to express themselves emotionally so easily.

The Masculine Prefers to Think

Men, being more fiery and head/thinking oriented, are much better at thinking things through on their own and tend not to need to communicate and relate so much. I think this is why the man-shed is so popular. Thinking an issue through to solution is very satisfying for a man and this leaves him feeling empowered and free – both vital experiences for the masculine whether in men or women. Women tend to need to talk things through and relate in order to get to solutions. Women, and men themselves, tend to give a guy a hard time for his inability to match her relating skills. Due to the rise of the "nurture over nature" theory, boys and men often feel shame about their alleged "communication issues" which women tend to point out. Men see that their masculinity seems to cause women a lot of trouble which can feel fundamentally painful and confusing for a man who is naturally hard-wired into pleasing the feminine.

He Thinks and She Talks

Men generally want to make women happy and so feel a sense of failure when they can't do it. We tend not to hear about this pain in men because communicating about "how we feel" is part of the feminine power of relationship. So the women talk about how they feel about all this "poor communication" and how their man isn't good enough and the men often go silent and think their worst thoughts. Men will hold onto stuff for years and never share with anyone the deeper things that trouble them. Whereas women will tend to natter to each other all the time about things that are on the mind. I heard Esther Perel – the famous couple's therapist - say once that in her work with couples, she invites the man to speak first as this is often the first time he has spoken. A man who is healing himself will naturally find relating with others easier as his inner feminine awakens.

Running Water Clears Itself

You see, women are like Earth, and as such are also watery in nature. When we communicate, we are like the babbling brook; in the same way that running water clears itself, we flow over each stone and we flow around each rock. If each stone were a possibility, our talking touches each stone to consider it. In this way, by touching each issue and by babbling like the brook, we get clear. Men tend to think to get clear and women tend to talk to get clear. Men like it when we ask them questions that support their thinking.

When a woman wants to relate about something deep, some men will interrupt in order to fix things. The fire element is about "doing" and so this is what he will do. He may need help to understand that in hearing us this is actually helping things. He will need some help in making that connection. Men want us happy and they will certainly attempt what we ask of them if they believe this will help us.

Men Like Clear Instruction

How many times have we heard a man say, "Just tell me what you want form me"? Unlike women, men tend to like to get clear first *before* they speak. When in relationship, they like to get to the point straight away – think solar flare or sword; sharp and clear. Even my own son, who has been brought up to relate well, has said to me, "Mum please can you get clear before you speak?" I was staggered when I heard him say this. I then of course "enlightened him" about the babbling brook feminine way. But as I was doing so, I realised that this situation was as much about my being *clearer* and honing my own inner masculine as it was about him making way for my feminine. He just needed me to verbalise what was expected of him (fire element) rather than have a long conversation using *him* to help me get clear (water element)! Thanks to his feedback, I took a breath and got to the point more quickly and he was able to be more patient.

He Has to Find His Own Way

If you live with a man, you may have noticed how he might resist doing things that you ask him to do? And how he doesn't perhaps do what you suggest? You give him advice and he gives you that look. You suggest he squash the milk cartons before putting them in the bin, but, there they are in the bin fully inflated and the bin is full far too quickly. And you ask him to do the work surfaces after he washes up and - lo and behold - not done or not done "properly". Here, a woman feels powerless and he feels trapped; and the feminine power of relationship is lost in the pain.

Your women friends' response to your housekeeping requests would be very different, thus horribly confirming that he is a stubborn so-and-so. Your women friends would "nest" right alongside you doing things in your home the way you would like them done; or maybe they would show you another way. But your man? No. Your helpful advice actually disrespects his masculinity, just as his unsolicited advice about your cooking might offend your femininity.

Feminine and Masculine Needs

Both the feminine and masculine have their own gifts and sensitivities, and being "advised" or told what to do is one of men's great sensitivities. Women have other great sensitivities. Learning to use our power of relationship can influence our man to become the knight of our dreams. He gets to then serve the feminine and be a hero and he gets a testosterone release from the action – and, believe me, that feels good for us too.

Learning how to use the feminine power of relationship is key to having a peaceful relationship with our husband or male partner, or for that matter, a son. Telling him what to do and constantly asking him to do stuff is not using your power well. It is controlling him, nagging him and not respecting his God-like Shiva nature. And so, becoming the Goddess that you really are and learning how to relate and communicate with him, will help your relationship. And believe me, this can be quite an arduous journey for some women.

Men Don't Like to Relate as Much

Although the masculine does like an intelligent conversation and is a sucker for debate, when it comes to emotional conversations and real relationship, he may find he has limited capacity. Torn between wanting to please his lady and yet withdrawing to the hills, he might stay and do his best. Men tend to be more expert at practical intellectual discussions and they tend to get quite stressed once a woman gets going with the many varying depths of discussions that she may tend to be more skilled at.

"What Are You Thinking?"

And then there is the "thinking thing". There he is sitting quietly at the table or on the sofa with you and we ask him, "Watcha thinking?" And he panics as his answer is "nothing"; or something that you might not want him to be thinking. "How can you be thinking about nothing?!" we may ask; "How is that even *possible*?!" We genuinely don't understand as we wish we could think of nothing, but it's never happened yet. We might then suspect him of thinking about something that he doesn't feel safe enough to share with us; thinking about how he doesn't really love us, about another woman, or thinking about how unhappy he really is proving that he does in fact need therapy or that he has got a psychological problem. Whereas he may well be quite okay actually, and just sitting, gloriously, being like the Sun and thinking about *nothing*.

We find this hard to believe, as when he asks us what we are thinking and we tell him "nothing", it usually means we are in deep pain and he is in deep trouble. We don't understand because we women are like Earth; we are so creative and hold so much and we are always busy and doing several things at once and our thoughts are relentless! We would *love* it if we could think about nothing! But men are like the sun and often think about nothing and I believe this is why men perhaps find meditation easier.

Never Trust "Ahuh"

Mark Gungor, again, who helps thousands of couples across the USA, talks about how men will be watching a screen and saying "Ahuh" in response to the very important communication that his wife is making. Gungor says how we should never trust any "Ahuh" a man is saying unless he is sitting and looking straight at us. As masters of relationship and communication we forget this because we can hold a conversation about something even while checking emails. (I can't personally do this but I have found most women can.) We think he is doing the same. Gungor says he isn't. He has *trained* himself to say "Ahuh", as he has found that this keeps his lady happy. I'm smiling as I type this. Many a time the guys are so keen to see us happy that they end up annoying us and genuinely don't understand how that all happened.

He Is Not Your Bestie

The many different ways of communicating all have their advantages. But as women, the power of relationship is honed when we work with *how* we communicate, and this is where we have a lot to learn – especially with communicating with men.

Remove Truth and Add Honesty

You see, women have been so busy telling the truth, and being "empowered", that we have disconnected from our power of *influence* which is often even more powerful! How ironic is this? As women we are incredibly influential but only if we communicate in an influential way. If we are just downright "truthful" all the time, we won't necessarily be influencing. Truth in itself can be brutal and biting and, ironically, rarely useful. "I think you are fat," might be a truthful statement but will not bring what you dream of. "I do find very healthy men sexy," whilst truthful, has an honesty about it that is more likely to influence your man to get off the sofa and into the gym.

In the polarity relationship, men can quickly get our back up by not speaking to us in the right way. And likewise, men are easily hurt if they feel disrespected or rejected. Men are particularly sensitive to feeling disrespected. Men and women are different and have different needs when it comes to how they want to be communicated with by their sweetheart. For example, we women might like to be spoken to in a particular way so that we get to feel feminine, sexy and open-hearted. And guys need to be spoken to in a particular way so that they can feel masculine, powerful and heroic. We don't feel wonderful when we are treated like a bloke and they don't feel magnificent when they are treated like a girly.

Enter, Radical Honesty...

Kim Anami's relationship and sex tips involve "Radical Honesty". This heart-centred way of communicating introduced into a relationship can be a real game changer if it's introduced in a gentle and respectful way and with the agreement of both partners. Creating a safe and maybe sacred space to both share things that have been on your mind that, although painful, if left unsaid could jeopardise the relationship, is in fact a very caring thing to share as it is actually protecting the relationship. Maybe one of you would like a bit more adventure in the bedroom. Maybe one of you has a pattern or tendency that is beginning to

160

grate. Maybe there is a dynamic within the relationship that is becoming frustrating. These might be painful things to hear, but if said for the betterment of the relationship and expressed with vulnerability and tenderness it can bring you closer together and can build an incredible level of intimacy. These radical shares can deepen a relationship and bring instantaneous re-connection overnight and even incredible sex. Of course, there is the element of risk, but this is the nature of vulnerability and true relationship. There has to be risk in it, otherwise it's shallow.

Deep Honesty Makes Deeper Intimacy and Better Sex

When we connect deeply with radical honesty to each other, our hearts expand and this brings incredible connection with amplified polarity - aka chemistry - in the bedroom. The heart is the positive pole of the pelvis and so when one pole is open and "charged" the other pole is affected. I remember my Tantra teacher saying that in helping thousands of couples with issues in the bedroom around vaginismus and lack of libido and lubrication, he has found that it is always to do with something going on in the heart. Always. No exception.

Real Relating Brings Peace and Happiness

When we move into our power as women and really use the power of relationship, the world ends up a happier place. The feminine tends to find it much easier to attune with the individual person they are with. A woman may have many children but she will know the different ways she will need to respond to those children in order to get the best from them and for those children to get the best from themselves. A woman in her feminine powers knows how to influence her man rather than control him. She knows how to relate with him in order to get the best from him and for him to feel like a king and behave like a hero.

Men Love the Chance to Have a Good Ol' Think!

Men like to work stuff out for themselves and they feel powerful when they do this. Here is an example of the power of our influence and the male need for respect. This is from a personal memory of Reid Tracy – the CEO of Hay House publishers. He's given me permission to use this. It was a conversation between him and his wife that I received in a Hay House email that I had subscribed to. Now some of you might find this difficult but I invite you to simply notice this, and see what happens for you as read on. The thing to really "get" here is that both of these people ended up *happy* at the end of the interaction. Reid writes:

"...I was excited to tell my wife Kristina that I'd agreed to buy the boat, as we'd talked about it for a few days.

I told her the news and she said "That's great! If you really want it and have thought about everything that owning the boat entails..."

Kristina fell fast asleep but I laid in bed tossing and turning, thinking over and over about the boat purchase.

After about five hours of no sleep, I got up at 4 AM in the morning and emailed Gordy that I'd changed my mind, because I "knew" that my intuition was telling me not to purchase the boat...

...As soon as I laid back down after sending that email, I immediately fell asleep.

When Kristina woke in the morning, I told her what I'd done.

She agreed, saying it was probably the right decision to cancel, as she'd come up with many of the same conclusions. But, she wanted me to have the boat if I really wanted it so hadn't shared them.

It's now two weeks later and I'm so happy I made the decision to cancel the boat purchase... things have worked out much better than buying our own."

This is a *happy* relationship. It's a fabulous example of feminine power. What she did was get him to ***think***. She wanted him to feel empowered and so got him using his own thinking processes. She didn't try and control.

Help Him to Think

Isn't that subtle? She got him using his head and men really need this. Men feel empowered and more masculine when they have thought something through for themselves and they feel respected when they are enabled to do this. In the case above, no one felt unheard or patronised. Everyone was happy. You see, guys being so fiery need the feminine to keep them cool and enable them to make good choices. Men are so fiery and focused they can end up making quick decisions and miss things. Because men are so focused and directional, they sometimes need a bit of help to slow down and think things through. Just as male fiery presence and clarity helps women when we get lost in one of our complex issues. In the situation above, she enabled him to think about what he wanted. I guess if she, too, really wanted the boat, the conversation would have been different; but she wasn't bothered about it and so wanted to empower him to make his own choice. Men really respect this and it opens their heart to their woman. She didn't interfere with his decision-making ability - which is a masculine power – and thus, her being fully in relationship with him enabled him to feel more masculine and the polarity of their relationship was nicely charged.

"Hang on a minute!" you may cry. Isn't this "mollycoddling" and "treading on eggshells"? Well, there are two answers to this. No and yes. No, because actually, it is just us practicing to use our power well, as men need their woman to use skilful words when they are having a challenge or when they are unsure what to do. And yes, it is also walking on eggshells which is sometimes what men have to do around their woman! He has to say the right thing in her time of need. It cuts both ways. It's how we love each other more.

Biding Time Gets Results

Like a hen sits on her eggs, the feminine knows how to bide her time to get the best results. There are times when she needs to be more forthright but this is a skill and she must be patient and wait for the right time. Here is an example of this with Marti, who finally speaks to her 19-year-old son after waiting for a year or more. This is typical of the strength and containment of the feminine:

Marti and Her Son...

Marti had been painfully observing her son get bogged down with his first girlfriend who had been diagnosed with depression. The girlfriend took medication for it. He wanted to be with her, especially for who she was *in between* her bouts of darkness. But when she was triggered, she would spend most of her time in bed – often days. She wasn't interested in trying anything to heal herself on any level and by the end of the year the dear boy was depressed himself. Marti held her tongue, knowing that she had to be careful – because of polarity – that she might unwittingly push her son further into the arms of this girl he felt protective of.

He finally began to talk about it to his mum while they were driving somewhere together and he described how he didn't want to hurt this girl he loved by leaving her. A dilemma for so many males. My friend could hold herself no longer, and responded, *"But does she do all that she can to become her **best self**?"*

164

On a daily basis, *is she doing **all** that she can do*?" And she said no more. The rest of the journey was in silence. It would have been so easy for her to go on and on here. But Marti leaves her son to think about what she just asked.

Marti's son evidently thought about what she had said, as by the end of that week he had ended the relationship.

In these two scenarios these women *got the guy **thinking*** for himself. There were no "helpful suggestions" or "advice". Nor was there control or manipulation. Just a wish for them to think about ***what they wanted*** and what they were about to take on or had taken on. Neither of these men would resent the woman they were confiding in.

Mike's Lack of Communication

My dear friend gave me permission to use this next example. Let's call her Rhianna. She was saying how Mike, her partner, was still very "passive aggressive" with his communications. I was very curious and she explained more: At her home, she had been in the kitchen that morning and had turned to Mike and asked what his plans were. She despairingly told me, "All he said was that he had a meeting today and that he needed to make space for that!"

Now, I felt a bit confused here as you might too. She then said she felt hurt and angry. I was more confused and even more curious. I suggested that his response sounded like a good match to her question. I went on to say that she obviously hadn't had her needs met though, otherwise she would have been okay and there wouldn't be an issue. I asked her what she needed that she hadn't got from Mike's response. "Well to me... " she said, "... when I ask him about plans in that situation it's to do with who's picking the kids up and who's driving whom where!" (They live in a village with teenage kids.) She felt very despairing of his "lack of communication and selfish behaviour" and was feeling dismayed and fearful about their future together. But I could see what had happened...

"It's a polarity thing," I said. "Men think and communicate in a totally different way to women." She had asked what his *plans* were. He told her. Job done. Ask a woman the same question and she might even engage you in a conversation for a while. But ask a man and he will be direct and to the point like a solar flare. Most men are very literally like the Sun - what you see is what you get. Men will assume that women are being direct too. In the example above, Mike was answering Rhianna's question. And he might have even felt pleased with himself that he could answer it so clearly. He had planned a meeting! Result!

Free Your Fire – State Your Preference

BUT what she *really* needed was *clarity about the family's transport arrangements*. She didn't want to know about his plans at all! "Think penis," I said. She laughed. It's pointing in a particular direction and some direction was needed here. "Please will you pick the kids up," is bossy and not respecting his Sun-like force. "Honey I'm thinking about the school pick-up arrangements. My preference is for you to do it?" might have done the trick. Here Mike would get to use his own brain which makes him feel more potent, and he gets to choose if he wants to be a hero in this moment which they would both benefit from.

She would be really smashing her feminine power of communication if later on, after our discussion, she found Mike and said, "Darling, I realise I wasn't clear this morning when I asked you about your plans for the day. I actually needed to let you know that my actual preference was for you to pick the kids up. Sorry about that." When a woman uses her power in this way her man would likely feel consumed by love and desire for her.

166

Relationships Trigger Our Trauma

Relationships trigger our trauma. They are meant to, as this
is how we develop as human beings. If our traumas are never
triggered, we would never get the chance to heal and develop.
If we don't ever want to have our trauma triggered then we are
best to not have a relationship and then not have kids either
because both of these things push us into development and
into reaching a higher state of consciousness. In the instance
above with Rhianna, her mother was not very attuned to her
needs and so when Mike was not particularly well attuned to
her either – she becomes triggered into these very early feelings
of deep disappointment and despair covered with her fiery
masculine fire to protect her heart. There is a lot of healing
potential in these moments for her.

Good men do want to hear what their lady needs. They really
do. They have a deep sense of service toward the feminine
that women do not quite understand. These guys *want* to
make their lady happy. They *want* to get it right so that their
lady can be delighted. When their lady is unhappy they
blame themselves and they turn inwards. We see this with
defensiveness or "stonewalling".

Why We Live with Men

When women connect with other women it's naturally very
different. Women often inherently sense what the other
woman needs. Just as men tend to know what each other
needs. But men are so different to us. With the tribe gone, we
tend to live with men and not other women. This is actually
a huge ask and polarity suffers. The gift of this arrangement
is that we can learn more about how polarity works and we
can find ways of increasing the polarity. For example, we can

make sure that both she and he have their own spaces in the home in order to express their own femininity and masculinity more fully. Spending time apart when things are good as well as when things are challenging is also another way to increase polarity and "charge". Living with our men, within a growthful relationship, can enable us to understand each other much more deeply and intimacy can blossom and the heart can open more...

Learning to Clarify Our Needs

As part of protecting the polarity in a co-habiting relationship, both women and men often need space alone in the house by themselves – but this is especially true of women who, in having a womb, very much resonate with the home and often need to nest. We might suggest to our man that we "need some space in the house to ourselves"; another woman would instantly know what that means. She might even sense that we needed that before we sense it. But men don't work that way. To many men, that statement of "needing space" doesn't really mean anything – it's too vague. So, to a guy we'd need to say, "I need to be alone in the house for a couple of hours today. How would that be?" This enables real relating as opposed to the more cloaked "Isn't there a job you need to do round at so and so's?" or, "Please can you take the kids to the park?" or worse, "Please can you go out?"

"Do You Need to Pee?"

Women are often so busy looking after everybody else that it can take her *ages* to discover what she really needs in any moment. Women tend to hint at what they need and it perplexes men like crazy as they tend to just say what they need. Tony Robbins was talking about this in one of his videos; he was teaching a young lad how to respond to a lady whom he might be driving along the freeway one day. At some point she might ask, "Do you need to pee?" Tony asked the lad what his response to that might need to be. There was some conversation and some teaching. Finally the lad got it right; "Ah!, do *you* need to pee?" The audience cheered. Tony congratulated him. The lad beamed. But the best bit for me was when Tony then enthused to all the men in the audience, "Yeah! So then you make it *happen*! You just turn off at the next junction and make it happen for her!" I fell in love with Tony in that moment.

Yes, men do also need to learn how to read their lady's subtle cues, but women need to learn to pinpoint their own needs too.

Non-Violent Communication

Men can get frustrated by our lack of clarity and our need for them to be as responsive as our female friends. They will never be able to do that. Men can feel incredibly relieved when we become clear about what we *really* need. Conflict happens when a need is not being expressed or therefore responded to. The late Marshall Rosenburg and his work of *Nonviolent Communication* (NVC) is perhaps THE BEST strategy and a treasure to find for conflict resolution, and I cannot recommend it highly enough. Marshall's magnificent and gentle fire clearly guides us to know about the importance of clear communication of our vulnerability and need, with as much empathy as possible, and how we can use this method with great success to bring more peace. You can find a full three-hour video of his San Francisco workshop with Marshall himself on YouTube, which I would recommend over any book on the subject. Here is a little teeny summary highlighting the main principles and what I have found to be the most important points.

NVC is Only for Conflict

If you don't know NVC then it's not what you might think it is. It's not just about avoiding swear words and being respectful. It's a very specific way of communicating in a conflict situation that arrests conflict immediately. **And NVC is specifically for conflict. If you try and use NVC in normal life for regular conversations and connection you will go crazy for sure, as will your loved ones.** This is really important to understand and may be why this technique isn't as well-known as it could be. In everyday interactions I regularly use the "cloaked accusation" words but when there has been a big difficulty, out comes NVC.

A Feeling or a Cloaked Accusation?

Central to the NVC method is learning to become very clear about what "a feeling" actually is. And for NVC to work we have to temporarily suspend the way we usually express ourselves emotionally. This might sound simple but it's actually quite a challenge. We have all heard or exclaimed things like, "I feel disrespected" or, "I feel attacked." Well, in a conflict situation, if the relationship is already ruptured, these statements create further conflict. These two statements are not communicating a feeling at all, but are cloaked accusations. In a conflict situation, when people's fight and flight system is activated, these kinds of statements are perceived as an attack and so take the relationship even further into conflict.

Vulnerability

True feelings expressed in a neutral way have the opposite effect as they are coming from a chosen state of vulnerability. True feelings are experienced physically in the body and we have to be feeling vulnerable in order to express them. This very act – of choosing vulnerability – creates *connection*. This very expression is what melts conflict. It's true feminine principle. And it is courageous!

170

Cloaked accusations	True feelings
I feel threatened/	I feel hurt/
judged	shame
abandoned	fearful
rejected	afraid
ignored	frightened
violated	confused
invaded	frustrated
unseen	sadness
unheard	grief
unloved	numb
unmet	bemused
attacked	dismay
disrespected	overwhelmed
exploited	despair
used	hopeless
	angry (NB anger and irritation are what we feel to cover the vulnerability of everything else on this list.)

Human Needs

The next level to NVC is regarding human needs. Human beings naturally want to respond to another's human needs. It is the way we are wired. If, from a state of vulnerability, we can express our deepest needs, the other is more likely to respond in their natural human way – to want to give.

So instead of saying, "I feel attacked," we might say, "When you speak to me like this I feel hurt and afraid as it is important to me to feel a heart-connection with you, especially when we disagree." This admittance of vulnerability and expressing a deep human need is much more likely to get a connecting response.

Empathy not Sympathy

If the argument continues it's because another vital NVC component is missing – empathy. Empathy is not the same as sympathy and the difference is crucial in any relationship but especially when we are in conflict with someone. Sympathy is not so useful as it's more about separating ourselves from the other's experience – even putting ourselves above them in some way and perhaps feeling a level of pity for them. But empathy is where we use our energy to deeply connect with the other person so we can *feel* how they *feel* in order to mirror them. This has a healing effect and can be transformative. Empathy is when we truly engage with the pain of the other person in order for them to feel truly heard and understood. It's a very powerful thing to do and it's a powerful thing to experience too. The Native Americans say that empathy is about "putting on another's moccasins". Sometimes we might have to really concentrate to do this and even say, "Ooh... 'scuse me a minute," (as we close our eyes) "... I'm just trying to feel how you feel so that I can understand you better." This is immediately disarming. Having done this, we might then say, "I can feel that you feel really hurt?" or, "Do you feel embarrassed/frightened?" (Notice the question rather than a closed statement as this helps keep everything open). When we do this, it helps the other person to feel deeply heard and "met" and that you are "on their side". This not only helps them to process how they feel but also tends to elicit a vulnerable response from them rather than an attacking one.

Using Our Body as a Gauge

Essentially, when we are in relationship with another, our own body can show us how the other is feeling as well as how we ourselves are feeling. On many levels we are not separate! Really, we are like antennae and we receive information all the time. For example, our friend might have shared something and we feel fear in our stomach and we may say, "Golly yes, I felt fear in my stomach when you said that." Or she might say about something else and our spine goes rigid and we can say, "Wow, when you said that my spine went rigid." We can actually use our own body to gauge what is going on for the other. This doesn't always work as we may ourselves have been triggered into feeling an old feeling and inadvertently project that onto the other person. Projection is very powerful and this is why it's so important to heal our traumas, as the more we heal, the more expert we become at differentiating what emotional material is ours and what is another's. It still can get muddled, which is why it's best to stay open and curious and ask questions rather than insist. Our bodies really are amazing when we use them this way.

Some of the NVC statements might sound contrived and you may feel uncomfortable when you first use them. But they can and do arrest an argument quickly. To simply attack and avoid vulnerability may well be easier and even more "natural" depending on what your upbringing was, but this new way will bring you more peace. It just does feel a bit awkward at first.

Vulnerability Heals

I guess it's the good news and the bad news that it is *vulnerability* that arrests an argument. Good news because there is a way to resolve conflict and bad news as vulnerability is more painful to feel than defensiveness. But when we express real feelings and real needs, human beings are hard-wired to respond in a human heart-centred way, rather than a human survival/threat-brain way. NVC brings us into the true power of the feminine – relationship.

Just to restate: Mr Rosenburg's full three-hour NVC workshop in San Francisco is available on YouTube and I highly recommend viewing it.

The Power of Two

I'm moving away from conflict now and looking more at general problem-solving. Two people in relationship with one another can resolve *anything*. With communication, hearing and grounding and an intention to be wise and resolve the problem, it's amazing what can be resolved and what solutions can be realised when two people get together. I say two people rather than three or more because once we get to three or more, we enter into "group dynamics" which is a whole other ball-game. Relationship is two people. With a group of three or more we are easily triggered into our childhood familial patterns of behaviour from our family of origin, and we naturally lose touch with the creative force that is available to us when we relate with just one other. Any problem can be resolved with two!

Anything Can Be Resolved with Two!

There have been so many times when I have used this power. Any more than two people and we are then into "group dynamics" which is a very different thing and is a completely different dynamic than the power of two. I have experienced two people resolving all sorts of things. I think of moments when I've been with my sweetheart or a friend and we have been wondering about a certain issue, and we determine to stay with the issue until it's resolved. It works every time. I remember when a friend of mine was so concerned about her very poorly grandson. There was so much fear. But we were determined to stay in relationship and on the phone until we had got to the bottom of *why* he was having the particular symptoms he was having and why he was having this *now*. Once we got it, the shift was tangible as the energy changed within us and we were both covered in goose-bumps. Yes, her Grandson was still in hospital, but now she knew how to support him and his family on a much deeper level in addition to visiting him in hospital. I believe the saying "two heads are better than one" is an acknowledgement of this power.

In Relationship with Our Children

With the development of humanity has come our ability to use our power of relationship with our children in a way that can create a beauteous and harmonious home. Now, most of us don't manage this as often as we'd like, but it's still more possible than ever before as there is so much support available now. (Notice how the super ego may attack here by quickly reminding us of the time we didn't manage this!)

Work with the Brain, Not Against it

Research now shows us so clearly how the brain works and how important it is to have a good heart-connection in place *before* any corrective teaching can successfully happen with our kids. We now know that punitive and reactive parenting

175

actually *prevents* deep learning and in fact ruptures the adult-child relationship. There needs to be consequences but if these are dished out without a heart connection in place then the learning fails. With practice and a determination to maintain the heart connection, discipline can actually feel helpful to the child and supportive to the connection. I have found this new way of bringing up kids to be transforming. The invaluable works of Siegel and Bryson's *No Drama Discipline* and Faber and Mazlish's *How to talk so kids will listen and listen so kids will talk* (teen version also available) are, I believe, must-haves for parents. These works and many others are built on the principle that the child's brain has to be in a non-threatened state for any effective communication to reach them and for any resultant update to happen. Mix this parenting knowledge with Marshal Rosenberg's Non-violent Communication teaching us that all conflict and acting out is a ***tragic expression of unmet need,*** and we can really see the potential for humanity.

When Our Kids Get Hurt by Us

I want to just say please don't worry about how much you have damaged your kids. That sounds like a crazy thing to say, but the spiritual contracts between parents and kids are complex and this universe is even more complex with many factors to take into account. Our culture is an incredibly difficult culture to parent in. I see it as fragmented and still very broken with mothers constantly put in a very difficult position emotionally and financially. Considering how this culture is set up, we are doing astonishingly well. As long as we are committed to doing our best from *right now* and are taking 100% responsibility for what we do and feel and are committed to our growth and development then we are heading towards peace. Our kids heal as we heal. In the end, I believe, we are really all here to heal together.

Some Relationship Tips

- Checking you have a good connection to yourself (perhaps by taking a breath and feeling the pelvic bowl) before you connect with another.
- Checking that the contract of your romantic relationship includes a Growth and Development clause is a God-send and can be a game-changer. With this in place, all challenges and conflicts within the relationship can be attended to with a view to development and growth and can stop any "victim/perpetrator" consciousness from taking a foothold. This is so with friendships too.
- "What do you need?" is a brilliant question.
- "What do I need?" is an equally brilliant question. (If all we can think of is what we need *from* the other person or what we need the other person to do *for* us, then another great question is "Why? Do I need them to do this?" Here we can get to the deeper levels of what we are really needing...)
- Radical honesty is another game-changer, especially for our romantic relationship. Of course, you must agree with each other as to how honest you want to be. E.g. "Does my bum look big in this?" Kim Anami in her couples workshops speaks of "keeping the glass clear" between you using radical honesty, and how this is vital for any relationship to thrive.

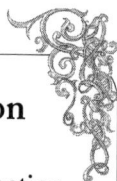

Relationship Prayer and Affirmation

You can adjust how you do this prayer and affirmation according to how much fire you need. (See Joy Prayer and Affirmation for more information.)
* I feel gratitude for the wonderful power of relating * I am getting better and better at relating * I make space to listen to my own needs * I verbalise my needs with ease * I easily recognise and state my preferences * I am open to hearing others' needs and preferences * I practice empathy with ease * I pause and listen deeply to the wisdom within my body * I'm able to help others become clearer about their own deepest needs * I forgive myself when I communicate poorly * I am willing to be vulnerable *

* I pause and listen deeply to the wisdom within my body * I'm able to help others become clearer about their own deepest needs * I forgive myself when I communicate poorly * I am willing to be vulnerable * ...

..."To nurture" is to assist someone or something to grow and develop over a period of time by enabling and nourishing and sustaining them on many levels.

Chapter 9
Nurturing

Nurturing

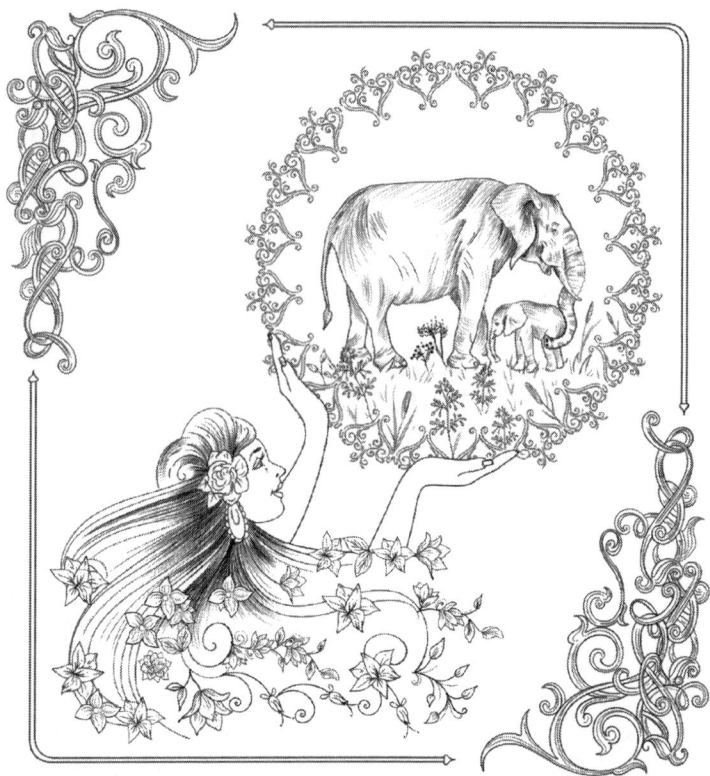

*N*urturing is how we assist someone or something to grow and develop over a period of time by enabling and nourishing and sustaining them on many levels.

Mother Nature herself is incredibly nurturing. She provides us with food and nourishment, constantly. Her waters cleanse us, heal us and her springs sustain us. Everywhere there is food. We have lost touch in this culture with what is safe to eat and prefer our things from the supermarket in packets, but the plentiful bounty is still there growing on trees and hedges and forest floors and meadows and orchards. Even grass is full of minerals and goodness and if not covered in pesticides can make a nourishing snack even for humans!

But she doesn't just nurture us with her food and water, she also nurtures us with her energy and she does this in two different ways: Attunement and Electrons.

The Attunement of the Earth

When we place our feet on the ground, or stroke the ground with our finger, the Earth plane "meets us" with equal pressure – with perfect attunement. If we take a moment to think about this, it's magical. Nature never gets it wrong. We are always met with equal pressure. Like a tender mother will meet the skin of her baby, so mother Earth meets us. She doesn't push with a greater force than you give. If you increase the pressure of your foot, she increases the pressure to meet your foot. It's like a game, only you'll never catch her out! Always perfect attunement!

Electrons

But Earth constantly emits electrons. Isaac Eliaz, M.D., M.S., LAc, the founder and medical director of Amitabha

Medical Clinic in Santa Rosa, California, says that when we walk *"...barefoot on soil, grass or sand, early studies are showing that the health benefits come from the relationship between our bodies and the electrons in the earth. The planet has its own natural charge, and we seem to do better when we're in direct contact with it.*

"A number of additional studies show how drawing electrons from the earth improves health. In one study, chronic pain patients using grounded carbon fiber mattresses slept better and experienced less pain. Another study found that earthing changed the electrical activity in the brain, as measured by electroencephalograms. Still other research found that grounding benefitted skin conductivity, moderated heart rate variability, improved glucose regulation, reduced stress and boosted immunity.

"One particularly compelling investigation, published in The Journal of Alternative and Complementary Medicine, found that earthing increases the surface charge of red blood cells. As a result, the cells avoid clumping, which decreases blood viscosity. High viscosity is a significant factor in heart disease, which is why so many people take blood thinning aspirin each day to improve their heart health. Another study in the same journal found that earthing may help regulate both the endocrine and nervous systems."

I'm not sure one could get any more nurturing than this!

The Feminine in Mothering

Feminine energy being so receptive and allowing is perfect for a baby's development. Nature knows what she is doing. You can drop into feminine energy and it will contain and envelop. The nurturing power of the feminine contains and cocoons like a chrysalis holds the cosmic soup inside it while it gathers itself together to form a butterfly. This "containing" can be hard and firm like the edges of a bowl holding your cereal in the mornings, or it can be soft and squidgy like your sofa at the end of the day. One thing's for sure. It's nurturing.

The Feminine Makes Space

A mother's feminine and magnetic energy naturally makes more space for the continuing incarnation and development of the baby whether born male or female. With his mother's energy, a baby boy has space to expand fully into his naturally centrifugal energy. And the baby girl with her super magnetic energy is then not overpowered by her mother's energy as she is just as receptive. So whether boy or girl baby, there is space for the baby's soul to incarnate more easily and more fully in the arms of the naturally receptive mother. We now know for sure that babies are calmed the more they are held by the mother or a female carer.

Mother Introduces the Ground

One of the tasks of a mother is to show her baby - through the bonding process - how to connect with the Earth plane. If the mother has a good connection to herself and to the ground, is *present*, and has a really good attunement to her baby, then baby automatically feels more connected to the Earth realm and will feel more nurtured and nourished. (If a mother was not able to do this, all is not lost, baby can learn to do this later on.)

Attunement *is* Nurturing

Attunement could be described as empathy, resonance and presence whilst responding to baby's need in the present moment. Attunement is now widely recognised as the most important ingredient in healthy bonding between mother and baby, and again latterly in any relationship - whether amongst friends or lovers or when caring for others' children. Attunement supercharges nurturing energy. To be well attuned, the mother needs to be relaxed and in her body. She needs to feel supported in her life so that she can be present in her body. From here she can make good eye contact, and equally sense when to give baby space. If mother can do this then she is a good bridge to Earth for her baby.

Connecting with Self and the Ground

No matter the beginnings with our own mother, we can now as adults attune to ourselves and the Earth, making our own connection. Then we can suck all that nurturing energy up through our feet and into our legs and into our womb or belly. As babies we are powerless and need to wait for our mother to make a connection so that we can then feel that via osmosis. But now we can take things into our own hands; we can now empower ourselves by making our own connection with our own self and with the Earth. We can imagine holding our teeny baby and ground down into Earth whilst holding her... and feel Earth nurturing us with her energy.

Trauma Affects Nurturing

Some women, due to wounds and traumas that they have suffered or bonded with in the maternal line, can find their nurturing ability affected by this. I have worked with women who have become more and more nurturing as they address old wounds in their hearts that had left them cold to the needs of children. When the feminine is of itself supported and nurtured, it awakens further. Men too, become more nurturing and loving when they tend to their wounds.

More Healing, More Nurturing

Some women can be incredibly nurturing even when their own childhood felt devoid of the nurturing that they needed. Here the woman seems to have an innate sense of what is needed as she knows more than anyone what was missing. It's as if in not receiving the nurturing she needed, she is now super sensitised to know exactly what's needed and can provide it, beautifully. She may get caught in nurturing others to the neglect of herself, but she will naturally nurture herself more as she heals her own trauma.

The ability to nurture; the softness of energy, the flowing of form, the sweetness or gentleness of voice, is bestowed to women in a way that leaves us turning to women in times of need. Whether we are male or female, if we find ourselves needing to feel nurtured, we instinctively seek out the feminine.

The Food of Women

We women exude nurturing to the extent that a meal cooked by a woman often just tastes better. It's what we mean by "home cooking" isn't it? Now please don't get me wrong and start e-mailing me about this. I have had some pretty amazing meals cooked by some amazingly talented men (my own included!) This has to be said for sure! But even many of those men when it comes to nurturing foods may well remember their *mum's* homemade soup or roast dinner or their *grandmother's* baking and so forth. I'm speaking about the nurturing power of the feminine that we women *particularly* embody and how this energy somehow imbues the food with this vibe. I'm smiling here as I remember a dear student who stayed with us for six months to learn English. His name was Gorkem and he was from Turkey. He and I were chatting in the kitchen and when I asked him what his favourite food was, he replied warmly, "Mother's sandwich." I smiled in my heart and gently corrected his English; "Oh that's lovely – your mother's sandwiches, yes..." And he corrected me with, "No, *any* mother's sandwich."

We Seek the Feminine for our Nurturing Needs

A man who is unwell will not turn to his mates for nurturing energy as he will not find it there, as men tend to teach each other and are more likely to insult each other. A man will naturally turn to us women for her power of nurturing not because he wants us to mother him but because he naturally seeks the softness of feminine energy. We women are the ones bestowed with the power of nurturing, the power of healing and the power of support (and so on) so it makes sense that our man wants to be with us when he is unwell or low. We ourselves might feel like he's our son and feel resentful about that – especially if we have had kids – but this is our projection. He'd much rather be your man than your child, believe me! (The latter would make him impotent so we know what he would prefer!) So his *need* for the feminine coupled with our innate nurturing energy does not make us his mother. It makes us his woman.

Men Generally Don't Want Mothering!

If we "fuss" over our man, he may well find this too mothering for him. He may well feel s-mothered and so push you away and feel grumpy. It's tough being a guy who needs support; too much support and he's back with his mother as a boy again and has lost his manhood. Here he then feels impotent. And yet without enough connection with his woman he will feel bereft. It's a tricky balance for a man. We women just don't have this issue at all! It doesn't matter how much support we get, we don't lose our femininity – we simply become more feminine as we surrender into it, but for men it can feel quite perilous.

Polarity Goes When He Is Unwell

But something does happen when our man is down on his luck or if he's unwell - the polarity gets messed up. A poorly man or a wounded man is not a fiery man. When he is down, he is not going to be our hero by taking us out on a date to awaken Eros tonight and we will not be melting in his arms anytime soon. Here we might have to "man-up" in order to take the slack and we can end up becoming over-tired and drained. The feminine after all wants to be shone upon! We want our man back! Or worse, if there is not much polarity in the first place – because he does not really show up as a man - then when he is ill, things feel as if there is no hope at all! At best we women feel sad as we miss him, and at worst we feel furious as he is gone – yet again!

So, if he is unwell and grumpy, we'll need to create some space so that we feel supported and energised and also to give him some space so he doesn't feel smothered. Here is when we can make some time to be with our pals! Tip: do this also when things are really good between you as well as this builds the polarity between you and builds magic in your relationship. This is also so for same sex relationships.

Breasts

Our wondrous breasts are the area of our body that most exemplify our nurturing power. Breasts are so nurturing that our babies and infants are easily soothed by them even if it is not "dinner time". I remember my good friend Joanne Barker who was a fabulous Doula saying to me that the breasts "call the baby's soul to incarnate more fully". She would encourage mothers to let their babies just lie on their bare breasts after and between each feed. This generally confirms to the baby that it was a good idea to incarnate. This makes lots of healthy brain connections for the new baby.

Men Are Captivated by Breasts

As the breasts so strongly express and symbolise nurturing and the full glory of the feminine principle we can perhaps begin to see why men are so utterly captivated by them to the extent that we women will never truly understand. Because we ARE the feminine, because we have these wonderful breasts we are at an advantage here. Guys don't have them! Unlike men, we never had to turn away from the feminine to find our self as a woman. Guys had to turn away in order to find themselves as a man and need to literally re-connect with the feminine in order to come back into their hearts. Ideally, they will make themselves an expert lover in order to guarantee them frequent and fine connection with us. To do this they will need to stay well away from pornography and find a wise source of information.

To Be So Separate from the Feminine

We women are so inextricably part of the utterly life-supporting and nurturing feminine that we cannot truly understand how it feels to be male; to resonate more with the Sun and be so separate from the feminine. Add this to the fact that men have such a strong connection to the fire element – and to the head and eyes in particular (which are the positive pole of the fire element) that they are very *visually* stimulated in a way that we women will never experience. Men are captivated by our beauty and by our amazing breasts. This does not mean that they are necessarily objectifying when this captivation takes them over (although that of course might be there additionally). It's more about understanding the visual impact the beautiful feminine has on men and in how we can respond to this. I'm not suggesting we allow inappropriate behaviour here! (Indeed, we need to keep the standards high – see Boundaries). I am suggesting that we find more understanding of polarity, and through this understand ourselves and men more. (Men are not going to be telling us what's going on for them – for this type of sharing is a feminine power and is more *our* domain, but what we can do is help boys - and influence men - to *ground* their energy so that they are masters of their sexual energy and not slaves to it.)

Self-nurturing

Self-nurturing is vital. It's vital as it *feeds* all the other things we do. And we respond with "Yeah, yeah.. I know..." and carry on reading, right? Well, we can't keep doing this. Not if we want to really embrace the delights of our womanhood and our femininity and change the world. Feminine energy involves us being alive and present in the delights of our body. The reality is that this takes certain self-care procedures to enable this energy. If we are exhausted, hungry, lost in our head and not loving ourselves then we cannot share our feminine energy with the world and we fail at femininity. Harsh words I know, but femininity needs nurturing. This is the nature of the beast. Consistently abandoning ourselves is a sign that there is trauma to heal. In my experience, we neglect ourselves if we were neglected on some level or if there was neglect in the maternal line.

Self-Care Empowers the Feminine

The feminine in general is suppressed worldwide, with the odd exception (as at 2023) and we see this with women trying to be everything and do everything. A life-coach was helping a woman who was married, had two little children, worked full-time and wanted to start her own business but "couldn't seem to focus". He suggested she cut herself some slack as the reality was that she actually didn't have much time. He suggested she currently focus on self-care. At which point she burst into tears as she hadn't realised that was okay to do. She thought it was selfish. This current culture totally leaves us thinking this way. But to be in our power as women we must reclaim our femininity and nurture ourselves so that we are "femmed up" in order that we are then powerfully effective in the world.

Some Nurturing Tips

- Women must nurture themselves first. For me, I include my alone time, my health and fitness, my sexual energy and my finances.
- What feels nurturing to you? Arrange that. It hugely enables us when we do something that feels nurturing to us. Every. Single. Day. Really. We have to really take care of this nurturing energy and fill up on it, in order to change the world.
- Our friendships need nurturing.
- I recommend Ann Wilson the Wealth Chef to help with nurturing finances. She is online and has a book called "The Wealth Chef".
- To nurture your sexual energy I recommend Sonja Maria Devi or Kim Anami – both on-line and have different styles of teaching.
- If I nurture my friends or family, I make sure I have the capacity to do so. I make sure I am full up first.
- I also practice letting my man give to me. This ensures I have energy to give back to him. I practice allowing in and letting go of control. If he asks what I'd like, I practice stating my preference but I also am learning to trust more; so I let him cook me a meal that I'd prefer another way, I let him put things away in the wrong place and I let him make the bed poorly. I have learnt to receive the intention and let go of perfection (most of the time).
- If my family is struggling, I might make a favourite family

meal. I don't underestimate the power of this. I have used this power very successfully.

- Kids need hugs. If we weren't brought up with hugs this may not compute but we can start slowly. I read somewhere that teenagers need twelve hugs a day to support their emotional and physical development. If our kid is not very "touchy" then we can start very slowly, respecting their boundary with a quick pat or stroke on the shoulder with no eye contact. Don't linger. When they feel safe enough, they will begin to soften.

Nurturing Prayer and Affirmation

You can adjust how you do this prayer and affirmation according to how much fire you need. (See Joy Prayer and Affirmation for more information.) * Thank you for bestowing me with the wonderful gift of nurturing! * I feel gratitude for my nurturing energy * I regularly nurture myself * I nurture myself every single day! * I am so filled up with nurturing energy that is given to me by my connection to the ground and to the Divine * I am a very nurturing woman! * The power of nurturing is so strong in my being and I allow it to flow through me * I feel this nurturing energy in my breasts, my heart and my pelvis and I ground it at my feet * I embrace my loving and nurturing energy! * I can feel that I am indeed a soul, incarnate here on earth to nurture life around me! * I am free to nurture! * I am willing and ready to nurture so many things into life and into form and into completion and manifestation! * I honour this nurturing energy in me *now*! *Yes. Yes. Yes! *

I am free to nurture! * I am willing and ready to nurture so many things into life and into form and into completion and manifestation! * I honour this nurturing energy in me now! *Yes. Yes. Yes!*...

...The feminine heals. Her soft, nurturing presence heals all ills. There are, of course, many fine Medicine Men and male doctors and nurses across the land, but nursing and traditional healing methods have tended to be done by women.

Chapter 10
Healing

Healing

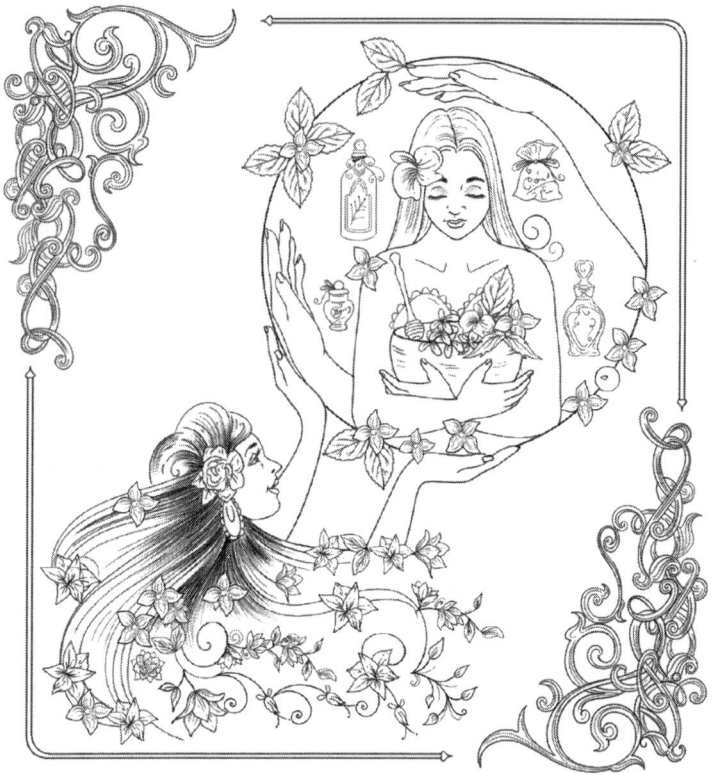

The feminine heals. Her soft, nurturing presence heals all ills. There are, of course, many fine Medicine Men and male doctors and nurses across the land, but nursing and traditional healing methods have tended to be done by women. Yes, we can see this as railroading or stereotyping; but if we only see it as this, then we miss another power of the feminine. We all know that when we feel unwell, we usually seek the feminine and not a bloke – no matter how feminine he is!

Wounds Seek the Feminine

Wounded children instinctively search for their mother or a female carer. As do grown men. We see this in the case of a medical orderly, dealing with grievously wounded soldiers, who said they would often have two requests. He could help them with a cigarette, but not with their mum. Even if our mother was more like a sergeant major, we would, whether male or female, still have longed for her when we needed healing or felt unwell. We will still need to be loved in a soft way.

We may well have longed for our father to love us in a warm way too, especially if he was too hard and cold. But in working with people over all these years I have found that with fathers, it was protection and warm encouragement and motivation that we needed from him, whether we were consciously aware of this or not. From our mother we needed softness, healing, nurturing and nourishment.

Nature is Self-Healing

Nature is always self-healing and developing. She fills cracks in tarmac and concrete with soil, grasses, mosses and flowers and she pushes up through our man-made mistakes with her tree shoots and herbs. I saw an image on Facebook of an abandoned ship covered in trees and vegetation. Even a war-zone will be healed by her strong, loving and nurturing energy eventually. Whether it's beautiful plant shoots growing up through lava or whether it is our errors that she is repairing, she does so constantly. In areas that were once incredibly polluted, life has quickly returned. Like the seal population in the river Thames in London. Otters have returned to our rivers and eagles and kites have returned to our skies. Nature's self-healing abilities are so phenomenal that she recovers quickly from our unconsciousness and from our experiments and mistakes – especially if we help her by our caring actions.

Humanity Amplifies Healing

Nature heals even more quickly if we bring in our human love to speed the process. She is very responsive to our healing intention and positive action. She is so responsive to us – because she is so feminine and receptive. We see this also with vegetables and plants that are actively loved and cherished; they can become huge and appear healthier and more beautiful compared to plants that are just left to fend for themselves and are just watered. A plot of land damaged by chemicals was given herbs and healing intentions and was soon full of worms again. A tree whose flowers were used to make healing flower essences now produces many times more fruit than the surrounding trees. We have not been told the truth as to the reality of nature and our power as human beings let alone the power of the feminine. As humans, we are all natural healers really and as women this is particularly so.

Exercise: A Woman's Healing Cupboard
- Dedicate one of your kitchen cupboards or a large sturdy box to be your Woman's Healing Cupboard.
- Gather things from around your home that help with healing - on any level - and put them in your new Woman's Healing Cupboard. Include all your remedies, essential oils and herbs and the like. Add in your favourite hot water bottle too and wheat-bags, even candles and incense... anything that gives a healing vibe for you.
- Consider "Marie Kondo'ing" the categories of products in nice little labelled boxes (with lids off for ease of grab) so that when you feel unwell the mere opening of the cupboard lifts your spirits and is a salve to your soul.
- When you've done all this to strict feminine standards of "That'll do", notice how you feel to have created this; "strong" "connected" "weighted" ... Say it out loud if you can (as this helps re-wire the brain). Then feel how you experience this feeling in your body (helps further re-wire the brain so that the feeling is "benchmarked").
- And that's it! You have powered up your feminine power of healing.

(Men have access to this power a little bit too, but don't usually feel quite so empowered from this kind of thing.)

Plant Medicine

Plants, flowers and roots all have their own unique medicine too. I have been staggered by the healing potential of everyday herbs and flowers just collected from my garden. Really, most of us have become so disempowered and do not take responsibility for our own health. Essential oils, too, have amazing healing qualities that are now very well-researched. I thoroughly recommend DoTerra as their protocols and research seem to be top-notch.

The common hedgerow is full of energy that we can use to heal ourselves. According to www.healthline.com, even grabbing a simple nettle leaf and letting it steep in a cup of boiling water is going to give us more than 22 health-giving properties and five other health benefits, with many others being a possibility! (In general, when using herbs, it is advisable to check with a qualified health practitioner if you have any doubts.)

Crystal Medicine

Every crystal has its own information within its structure, its own healing ability and thus its own unique "medicine". They are very powerful to use in a healing capacity. They are quietly used in our everyday technology too, bringing us life as we know it by the power their conductive energy.

Water Medicine

Even Mother Earth's plain water can be used for healing. It naturally flushes our system through and keeps us hydrated. It also keeps the blood cleaner and helps keep the bowel flushed and our skin clearer and so much more besides. Thanks to the work of the wonderful late scientist Masaru Emoto we can see how water is so receptive that we can even programme it with different intentions to help heal ourselves with it!

Healing Ourselves First

Women are so endowed with the natural power of healing - but we must heal ourselves first. I believe this is all part of the path to womanhood. But how do we heal our self? Well, that answer is a

book in itself and there are so many ways. Here are some things I
have learned along the way that have helped people.

- Grounding into the feet and sitting bones contains us and shows
  all stuck energy where to ground out – when it is ready to do so.
- Gentle belly breathing helps with transmuting emotions and
  processing old material. The fire of transformation does need a
  good supply of air; exhaling first to shrink your lower belly and
  then letting the breath "fall" in, filling your belly first, before your
  chest cavity. Softly...
- Use self-compassion when you are struggling and in pain or
  under super ego attack. Self-compassion puts body and brain in
  healing mode. If you can't feel self-compassion, try asking, "Why
  not? How come I don't deserve compassion here?" and see what
  comes up. E.g. "Well I should have sorted this out by now." Here
  you can ask, "Can I feel compassion for the part of me that hasn't
  been able to resolve this yet?" and so on until you get to a place of
  self-compassion. Self-compassion = healing mode.
- "Tapping" is a great method and resource and can be learnt
  online for free. I recommend the Tapping Solution developed
  by the Ortner family. This form of tapping has helped me
  enormously with my own embodiment, helping me to name
  feelings and where they are in my body. Tapping helps us to first
  accept how we are feeling emotionally in our being, even if we
  don't understand *why* we are feeling the way we do. It puts our
  body and mind into Self Compassion mode before we can then
  use this method to further help us to release stuck emotions or
  feelings from our body.
- I always see physical symptoms in our body as messages from
  a part of us that needs healing. If the pain or symptom had a
  feeling what would it be?
- Jade-egg work can really heal our relationship with ourselves
  and our feminine sexuality and is so central to our inner sense of
  peace and groundedness. Sonja Maria Devi does beautiful online

training and webinars on this.

- When we sense and track "negative" feelings and emotions in our body and rest our full awareness on our inner experience, the energy changes and can "ground out" or be transmuted, especially if we include sensing our feet. Ideally, we want to wait around long enough to feel some sort of heat in the area of the emotion or feeling, or in connected areas. This is your fire literally burning up the feeling and integrating it. You might hear your digestive system rumble as we digest emotions in much the same way as we do food.

- Overwhelming feelings, that you find yourself avoiding, need more support. Find a practitioner or a therapist who knows how to work safely with trauma (a definition of trauma that I use is that there is an old overwhelming feeling that has not been integrated).

- Embodiment. Transmute the trauma in your body and psyche (same difference) and you will feel more and more comfortable in your skin.

- Grab a pen and try the exercise below. It's a way of exploring what it means to our unconscious mind to be a woman. The answers can be surprising and let us know what we need to attend to. See if you can write the answers very quickly without thinking:

Being a woman means:

....

Being a woman is:

....

Being a woman is sometimes:

....

Being a woman is mostly:

....

Being a woman is always:

....

Being a woman is never:

....

Then, after a while of absorbing the sobering reality of your beliefs (and/or of the beliefs you have inherited from your family of origin and the culture we live in) you can then explore each statement further, checking also for truth, as the super ego does quite like to paint a much worse picture.

We Are All Transformers

As human beings, we are all transformers. We are all alchemists. The body can change energy from one frequency to another. It can change fear to love. It can change dismay to gratitude and fear into excitement. When we sense inwards on a painful feeling and bring our consciousness to it, we enable this transmutation to happen; and if we stay with observing it long enough, while breathing and grounding, we can be left with a different experience. When we live our lives this way, this can be a powerful preventive medicine.

What's Behind a Symptom

All physical symptoms have their very *physical* reasons for existing but it is now very well known that they have an emotional component too and I have seen this for myself over and over and over again! Healing our emotional wounds is par for the course if we want to really heal our psyche as well as our body. Even with the "common cold" that may be experienced by a whole family, each member of the family will experience the cold differently and have different emotional "stuff" that is being cleared out via the mucous. If some kind of illness is part of our dying process, transmuting the accompanying negative feelings as we go will make even *this* process powerfully transforming.

Where Is the Feeling in Your Body?

When we bring absolute, astute awareness to the physical sensation of a negative feeling – and perceive it there in our body, this changes it. Try it. Let your body show you what it can do! Next time you get triggered with old painful feelings gnawing at your system, see if you can name, quite distinctly, the feeling underlying it all and then see if you can sense into where this feeling tracks into your body. Rest your full conscious awareness there. Every now and then, feel the rest of your body too and tune into your feet and sitting bones to ground it out into the earth.

The Magical Mid-line

Usually, we can sense feelings and emotions in our mid-line from our throat down to our lower belly and right down to our yoni and anus which are right where the water and earth chakras are. For example, we might feel panic in our throat, love and connection or longing in our chest, anger or fear might be in our solar plexus and terror might be experienced in our lower belly, vagina or anus. But unprocessed emotions can be held anywhere at all in the body due to how musculature and the autonomic nervous system reacts to emotions and feelings. So our shoulders may feel tight or heavy, our legs might feel numb and our spine might be rigid and so on. Thoughts and imagery *about* the emotion are of course experienced in the head area but the work to be done is with *sensing*; sensing the actual physical sensation of the feeling.

Healing Ourselves and the World

When either men or women do this kind of emotional processing, we add to the critical mass phenomenon. This means that when we are doing this kind of transmutation – whether meditating or emotional processing – we are doing it for the whole world as well. We are all connected, we cannot ever just be healing ourselves. Humanity and energy don't work that way. Thus, our private and individual work helps the whole world. I strongly feel that healing ourselves is, in reality, an act of great generosity.

In the healing fields, there is a greater percentage of women in this work than men. Of course, as more and more men are freed up to choose work they love, this percentage ratio is changing and there are more and more men in the field. But there are still proportionally more women in this work and there always will be, for it is softness we tend to seek when we are off-kilter.

Why Am *I* Doing All the Work?

A common complaint amongst developing women who are in a polarity relationship is that they are the ones "doing all the emotional and healing work". As incarnations of the feminine principle and being so like Earth, one of our powers is the natural predisposition to development and healing. Guys just don't have this like the gals do! Men have an *inner* feminine so that they can just about keep up! But women are the leaders on Earth in this regard. And the more women develop, the more their loved ones are influenced by this and get to grow too. The feminine is so powerful in this way.

Our Bosom Is a Balm to All

As women, as incarnations of the feminine principle, we are especially endowed with these healing powers even if we have no sense of them at all. Our soft bosom simply is a balm to all and the tenderness of our touch simply is healing to others. So, like the baby boy with his exhausted dad. The baby was crying non-stop whilst waiting to board a plane and would not stop crying until he was against the healing bosom of the female passenger next to him. Here the feminine heals – like the Catholic nuns in the leper colonies in South Korea, never getting ill themselves. As if they are actually as Nature herself, moving round helping, supporting and healing. Her touch. Her love. Her support... Her wisdom ... here the feminine heals.

If you are a woman reading this, even if you have no qualification in "healing", please know that just because you wake up in the morning, you are a healer. Because you are like Nature herself, you have been born with this potential in your feminine being, and you are, potentially, very healing to be around. Knowing this, consciously, empowers you tenfold.

Some Healing Tips

- It can be incredibly supportive to find a mentor, therapist or coach to help hold the space whilst we heal. But if this is financially impossible, I highly recommend "Tapping" or EFT – Emotional Freedom Technique. It is easily researched online and many Tapping experts offer freebies.
- I like to remember that only part of us needs healing, the rest of us is okay.
- If you have a physical symptom, what is your body holding for you that needs healing? Ask your still small voice within your heart and upper chest area and then pause and listen deeply to the answer you are given.
- Can you feel compassion for how you feel?
- Explore Natural Medicine as this medicine deeply resonates with our multidimensional energy and leads to deeper and more profound healing.
- Did you think Grounding was just to do in emergencies?
- Fully healing ourselves can be uncomfortable. There is some pain to go through but the end result is worth it. We hear of something being "healing" and we perhaps imagine something feeling really lovely, perhaps like a soothing massage. And sure, a massage can feel healing, but my experience of healing is that it's a much more

dynamic and powerful thing and often very uncomfortable. It involves experiencing feelings that we had to disconnect from in childhood. But the wonderful thing about being an adult is to know that as adults, with the right support and done slowly enough, we can feel through just about anything we have experienced simply because we *survived it all.* This is vital to recognize. In the safety of adulthood, with the war now over, we *can* now feel feelings that, as babies or children, felt overwhelming. In this way, adulthood by its very nature is protective. With an adult nervous system and with us no longer dependent on anyone for survival, our adulthood is a safe place to begin to reconnect with ourselves and to digest that which we haven't been able to digest before.

Healing Prayer and Affirmation

You can adjust how you do this prayer and affirmation according to how much fire you need. (See Joy Prayer and Affirmation.) * Thank you for bestowing me with the wonderful gift of healing! * I lovingly heal myself! * I accept and love myself, even though parts of me still need healing * My body has all that it needs to heal itself! * My immune system is as strong as the Cosmos! * I recognize that I am not broken but just unfinished as yet * I notice I attract people into my life who help me to heal in some way * I notice I attract events into my life that help me to heal in some way * I recognise that life shows me what is left to heal by repeating situations until I have healed the wound * I can feel that I am indeed a soul, incarnate here on earth to heal myself and help others too! * I help the earth to heal too by connecting to her more and more *

I recognise that life shows me what is left to heal by repeating situations until I have healed the wound * I can feel that I am indeed a soul, incarnate here on earth to heal myself and help others too! * I help the earth to heal too by connecting to her more and more *...

...Support is everything. Without it we wither away or become so utterly defensive that we destroy ourselves. With the feminine power of support, we thrive in everything that we do. Support is arguably the most invisible power that the feminine has.

Chapter 11
Support

Support

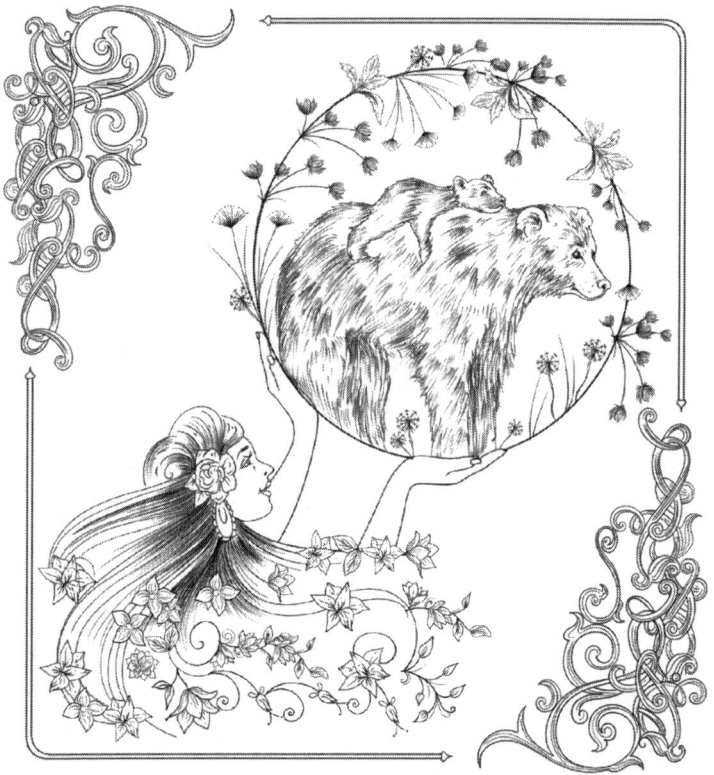

upport is everything. Without it we wither away or become so utterly defensive that we destroy ourselves. With the feminine power of support, we thrive in everything that we do. Support is arguably the most invisible power that the feminine has. For usually, it is the thing that is supported that is given credit and not the support that enabled that thing to happen. We see this in a theatre production; where the actors get the biggest and loudest applause but the pizza delivery boy who delivered pizza to the cast during rehearsal, even though he felt unwell and whose girlfriend has just left him, gets no mention. For he is invisible. The feminine is like this with amazing parts of us that are never seen. And, this is what makes the feminine, feminine. Such is life, we say. But let's look more at this power and see more of how amazing it is...

Trauma Prevention

Support prevents trauma. Full stop. Given the right support after a traumatic event, the body and psyche are often completely able to integrate the overwhelming event. As ordinary human beings we are able to do this with each other. If the support is not there, or if it's there but poorly attuned and out of kilter, then the energy of the event can't let go. For example, "suffocating reassurance" and "hysterical stroking" actually interrupt the body's natural ability to discharge energy and re-orientate after a shock. Spacious support afterwards from a loving human presence enables tears to flow and shaking to happen as the shock literally discharges out of the body.

Support After a Shock

Beatrice was knocked off her bicycle. She was bruised and cut but "okay" and got back on her bike and cycled to work. When she arrived, her favourite colleague and friend Amy was there and could see something had happened. Amy was concerned yet calmed herself by breathing deeply. Amy was then very present and gentle as Beatrice shared what had happened. Tears came for Beatrice and she found herself shaking and this was allowed to "ground out". Amy made tea for Beatrice and made one for herself too, and they sat together in a side office. Amy knew another colleague would have some Rescue Remedy and searched her out with success. After a long while, with this support, Beatrice eventually realised that she in fact needed to go home. A taxi came and took her and her bike home and she had a gentle restful day while her body integrated all that had happened. Amy phoned her in the evening to check how she was. Given space and loving support by Amy and her own self, Beatrice was literally able to let go of what happened and her wounds healed very quickly. Had Amy not been there, it might have been a very different outcome.

No Support Makes Trauma

If we don't get the right support after an overwhelming event, the shock and the associated feelings stay in the body and it then becomes a trauma that can get "triggered" later on. Luckily, this doesn't matter as we can then get support even years later and then release the shock at *that* point. With the feminine power of support well presented, in a way that is "just right" for the circumstance, the event gets integrated and we are strong once more to continue our life and are more *present*.

Support is Always Attuned

Support is what a person needs and not what we *think* they need. It is totally unique to any moment. "Rushing in" is rarely supportive. Pausing and sensing what may be needed is always supportive. Maybe a hand hold, maybe no contact at all, maybe a cup of tea and a blanket, maybe silence and peaceful observation. Maybe a gentle holding of the person so they can let go. Maybe just sitting next to them or making a phone call for them. All incredibly individual and unique to the person and the situation.

I believe that we won't need therapists in the future. Therapists are needed when support is missing. Therapists are needed in a culture that is broken; a culture that has been fragmented, that produces families and communities that are fragmented and disconnected and lost. It is the feminine power of support in therapists and coaches and in humanity itself which will heal all this fragmentation and enable wholeness and integration and a wonderful new world.

The Support of Earth

The Earth is incredibly supportive and so attuned to our needs! Of course, we have the company of the Sun, without which Nature would not be able to support us to the extent that she does. Unlike the Sun, her very physical support and nourishment are right there underneath us. And as we step lightly or push firmly into her surface, we can feel her gently meeting our weight with that ever-adjusting counter-pressure that she does so well. Here, Earth is always supporting and "under-standing" us in our current state of being.

When we stop and allow ourselves to tune in to the feminine power of support - and really feel this energy in Earth - we might notice that she never pulls away or gets fed up with us. She is perhaps our real mother whilst we live down here on our human journey. She has no judgement either. Her support is not conditional; she doesn't say, "I'll support some of you but not others." Her support is all-encompassing. No matter what we have done and no matter what we have experienced, she holds us.

How Actually Is the Earth?

If we listen to the current information that is being broadcast all around us, our sense of safety and that feeling of being supported by Earth will be compromised. Some may fear "tuning in" to Earth lest they discover that she is in such a state that they are not supported at all. This is actually a core wound for many people whose mother was not able to be supportive enough due to her own wounds. In fearing that Earth is damaged irreparably, we may become more ungrounded and more disconnected. But here's the thing, have you actually *asked her* how she is? Have you asked _Mother Earth_ how she is?

Ask Her...

On the Earth plane, there is lots of damage. There has been much destruction. Our culture has been one of over-consumption and pollution caused by plastic manufacture, toxic chemical production and electricity generation. Over-mining and road building have also caused a great problem. There is much healing to be done. _But..._ until we have actually asked how she is, we will not know for sure.

How might we do that?

Well, we might do it in the same way that we check in with a friend. When I check in with a friend, I ask verbally, yes, but I also sense in with my body. I *sense* how she is. This is how we can tell if our friend is not okay even if she says she is; our body senses will know the truth of it! If our friend says she is fine but we can also feel a sense of discomfort in our body then we know she is not really wanting to share right now. If our friend's response "tallies up" with how we feel, we know we are in true connection with our friend.

Feel how she is...

In the exercise below, I show you how you can literally *feel* how

Earth is. We can feel her response because we are also *part* of her. Just as we are connected to our friend and can sense and know how she feels, so we are connected to Earth and can sense and know how she feels too. It's all about energy and frequencies. Everything is energy and frequencies, and all is interconnected.

Here, as I ask mother Earth how she is, I take care not to *imagine* how she is. This might conjure up imagery that I have seen in the media that may have frightened me and that I may then project onto Earth. What we really want here is to create a *real relationship* with Earth in order to feel the truth.

Exercise: sensing how Mother Earth is

- So, take a seat and get comfy. Feel both of your feet flat on the ground. Please don't skip this bit. This is part of actually connecting with her. (This is the first step towards relationship; reaching out and making an initial connection.)
- Sense into your sitting bones…. Sense and feel how they connect with the chair underneath you. If the chair is soft this will be more challenging. But doing this, anchors you further.
- Then, begin sensing deep into Earth. Sense into her, there underneath you …. And all around you. And when you are ready…. ask Earth, "How are you?"
- Now *feel* her response in your body. Don't think. Feel and sense into *your* body, as this is where her response will be.
- She doesn't use words. She shows you in *your* body. This is how connected you are to her…
- What do you feel in your body? What is one word that would describe how you feel in your body right now?
- You might want to stay awhile, just feeling her response within you… It might take you a little time to name the experience as it will be using a different part of your brain,

---

but stay with it and find the words if you can and say the words out loud. This lets your brain wire-up this experience. Many women feel her response as a strong *weighted* sensation. It can feel both "solid" and "calm" and certainly okay.

- How does it feel to know that Earth is okay? Do you feel more supported?

As with any information about anyone, we really have to connect with that person, animal or entity ourselves in order to see how they *really* are. Until we do this, anything else is just hearsay.

When I do the above exercise with my clients, it can be a game-changer. Their whole universe can shift in that moment. You see, we need to take care of Nature, but not because "if we don't we will perish". We need to look after Nature because she is part of us and we are part of her. When we connect fully with her we align with the feminine power of support. When we hurt Earth we are hurting ourselves. Ever noticed the state of the men whose work involves clearing forests for new roads or new "developments"? They appear haunted to me. They have to disconnect to do it, and they suffer as they are attacking the very energy that supports them. This actually affects the soul and I can see this. When we are disconnected we feel unsupported.

Her Support Is in Everything Solid

Up to a point, the feminine power of support and the energy from Earth is in all physical things. We see this grossly overbalanced in materialism (mater/mother-ialism) where we have been sold on the idea that the more possessions we have the more supported we will somehow be. But in a more balanced way we feel Earth's support in all *structures* around us; we can feel Earth's support in any situation we may find ourselves in. Even if we are halfway up the Eiffel Tower, we can feel her support in the form of the iron and steel structure that we stand on... I always say to my clients - feel the energy of Earth *in the form of* the floor underneath you... and in the form of the chair at your back and under your bottom and under the back of your legs... and then often they breathe deeper... as they are back in touch with what supports them – their own body and its connection to Mother Earth – her huge, firm, supportive energising self that supports us throughout our Earthly journey here and she never stops supporting us... holding us – her child.

All Structures Are Supportive

All structure is an expression of the feminine power of support. This is true whether it is support from physical structures, or support by structuring a meeting, a conference or holiday or even our working day. Structures in their many forms support us, and, true to polarity, there are of course other structures in this world that do not support us at all - and this has been going on for millennia and is coming more to light at this current time.

"I Couldn't Have Done It Without You"

To use the example of Jesus, there is a theory that Jesus was only able to attain the levels that he did due to his relationship with Mary Magdalen. Many successful men and women will credit their very supportive wife or partner for their success. I see this dynamic all around me. The feminine power of support enabled many a man to do work which he might not feel able to undertake without that support in place. I think of all those men who spent torturous years down in mines and out at sea who would come home to dinner on the table. The feminine power of support has enabled many a child and teenager to come through mind-numbing schooling and through tough times as they explore their own life-choices and relationships. Of course, many women would say they could not do what they do without the loving support of their man.

Any system that supports is a manifestation of the feminine and its many incarnations of the feminine principle. "I couldn't have done it without you," is what so many supportive people hear.

She Supports and He Motivates

The masculine has its variant of support known as service, encouragement, motivation and enthusiasm. Also, that "getting stuff done" that men do. It is more dynamic and power-based – burning up more quickly than the cooler, more strong, heavy and steadfast energy of the feminine that tends to hold and contain all processes in a firmer and solid way.

The power of support contains us and holds us and enables all of the other powers. For support is needed for everything in our life. All of our powers and ways need support, our joy needs support, our creativity needs support, our pleasure needs support and so on. And it's the feminine power of support that enables our whole world to run smoothly. So keep absorbing Earth's amazingly supportive energy. Feel her supporting *you* dear sister... for she has supported you all along. It's just that you didn't know how to drink in her energy. But now you do. Through your feet! May you receive the support of the feminine right into your bones! May you feel re-charged and alive.

Supporting Ourselves with Self Care

Part of embodying the feminine power of support is about how we support ourselves. We can do this in various ways; physically, financially, emotionally, mentally, spiritually. Keeping our selves topped-up with energy by respecting our own needs and boundaries is vital to our health and to the health of our relationships and our family. This is acknowledged in the saying "If mama ain't happy... ". When we support our self by respecting our own needs, this also makes us a powerhouse for supporting others. If we keep abandoning our self by disregarding our needs, we may well want to support others; but if we do, we will be unconsciously taking energy *from* them. Years ago, I remember offering a dear friend a foot-bathing ritual. She accepted. A week or so later, she gave me some feedback that was hard to hear. You see, I had only just moved house a week or so prior to her treatment and through the ceremony she could feel just how much support I myself needed and so this spoilt the ritual for her. She found herself energetically "looking after" me, and so she was unable to really let-go into the treatment. This was vital for me to hear and I'm so grateful she told me and I hope in reading this that it helps you too in some way.

If there wasn't a highly-attuned and developed connection with our own mother early-on in our life, then self-support will be something that we have to determinedly seek and master in adulthood – otherwise we might always feel as if we are running low on fuel.

Physical Support

The feminine power of support is felt strongly when we have taken care to support ourselves physically with a nice-enough home, good-enough clothes, a healthy-enough diet, an income to support all this and plenty of time in Nature. Being or becoming financially independent is part of this as it brings us that empowerment that feels supportive. If you choose to not use money, building a repertoire of skills that can be shared is another way of supporting ourselves and "trading" this way can feel very satisfying. Having a good sense as to how to support our own health *naturally* is also part of this base layer of feeling supported. Dependence on patented drugs to feel well can leave us with a level of insecurity as any dependency does. Exploring ways of healing ourselves naturally is incredibly empowering and dynamically supportive!

Emotional Support

How we support ourselves emotionally is vital to our sense of peace and happiness. Of course, supporting ourselves physically is foundational to supporting ourselves emotionally!

If we have a history of lack of support, we might expect or depend on emotional support to always come from *outside* of ourselves, as is natural if our own vessel was not filled originally. This would be an old way of surviving. Or we might have survived the other way and become super self-reliant, fearing vulnerability, and letting no one in with an "I don't need anybody thank you" approach, or a mixture of both which is most common.

In health though, the adult is a self-supported, interdependent and *open* being. The adult can contain and process difficulties and challenges, and also knows when to reach out and connect with others and receive extra support when needed.

Self-compassion Is Vital

Another way of looking at this is that in health the adult self naturally supports the inner child. There is self-compassion for the inner experience during the trials of life. When things feel overwhelming there is an ability to receive support from others too where we might feel as if we have become the inner child. Later, I speak about support from others; but here I touch on self-support first and what that might look like as this is the most important relationship we will ever have: the one with our self. When we get this right, relationship with anyone else is always easier!

When Old Wounds Are Triggered

I see self-support and our relationship with our inner child as synonymous with one another. The inner child manifests as our playful, joyous and creative nature and also as our emotional pain and suffering. An aspect of our inner child expresses in us in particular when old wounds get triggered in the present moment. There we are, quite happy, and then woosh! There we are, in pain again, as if for the first time. The pain may be subtle or huge but there it is in our solar plexus, or heart or somewhere there... where it always feels a bit too big. We might be full of tears or find ourselves retreating within ourselves. Or we might get a headache or a "bad back" or any manner of symptoms that don't seem to connect to the present moment at all.

But I see all these emotional and physical symptoms as a communication from the inner child to us as the adult. Support is needed. It's when our inner young self is pulling on our sleeve in some way or has gone into shock and needs our presence.

Carrying on Regardless

And how do we respond to our self in these moments? How do we respond to these inner "communications"? Do we sit with our feelings and anxieties and feel them in our body and help them to process by breathing deeply? Do we feel compassion for ourselves and pause and sense inward to our inner pain and our inner world? Or, do we just try and carry on regardless? Who taught us to do this and how does it serve us now?

Self–attunement

Ideally, when we feel reactive or triggered in some way we pause and breathe... ground... We might put our hand on our chest and the other on our belly and we might verbally sigh and "coo" to our inner child in that soothing way that a very responsive mother might do until her little one is settled or at least soothed. We might put our arms around us or – even better – around a pillow that represents the wounded part (or a rolled-up coat will do) and we might say to our self, "Oooo... golly yes... that *did* happen and yes... it was SO painful, wasn't it..." We might look like a bloody idiot sitting there talking to our self this way but we can't worry about that BS when healing needs to happen. We have to *do* this! If we want to feel more supported then this kind of thing actually rewires the brain so that we *become* more supported!

If feasible and appropriate, we might then engage with what might comfort us further. Maybe we *can* then carry on, but with awareness of our little one in our heart or belly. Or maybe we need to snuggle with our inner self on the sofa or take a walk. Or maybe we can say to our inner self, "We need to stay here for a bit but can leave soon and head straight to the sofa / our friend's house / the bath / Nature."

Imagination as a Bridge

In these moments, I use my imagination as a bridge to my inner child. I "imagine" my inner child's response to the soothing words of validation and connection. I literally imagine her and see what she is doing and I trust that. She might not respond if I haven't got the statement right or she might snuggle in towards me if I have. Either way, I make time to explore.

Self-compassion Re-wires the Brain

When we respond to old wounds with self-empathy and self-
compassion, this prepares the brain and nervous system for
healing. According to the National Institute for the Clinical
Application of Behavioural Medicine, self-compassion is so
powerful that recent studies have shown that it even protects us
from PTSD after conflict situations in war zones! The studies
showed that servicemen and women who had an ability to be
self-compassionate were less likely to be traumatised after an
overwhelming event and were less likely to develop PTSD
nine months later. Self-compassion seems to create wiring in
the brain that protects the nervous system.

When we respond to our wounding with validation and self-
compassion, it is very integrating. We can change history in
these moments. Supporting ourselves like this is what it means
to live in a state of connection. It feels good!

Supporting Ourselves Spiritually

How we nourish ourselves spiritually too, is vital to our
health. Not in a religious sense although it could include
that for sure. I'm talking about discovering what deeply
nourishes and supports our soul. For me, this means doing
something that connects me with an experience of there
being some kind of higher power. It could be anything. For
me it's Yoga, uncovering/hearing great truths, sharing my
knowledge and understanding, getting outside for a walk in
all weathers, remembering it's a multi-dimensional universe
and I am a multi-dimensional being as part of that universe.
For someone else I know, it's quilt-making and prayer.
Another, it's making jewellery and walking her dog in
nature. More recently since March 2020, I have felt drawn

to the Christ energy in particular. (I gather this specific frequency is *particularly* useful and indeed most *powerful* in these current times.)

Support From Our Friends

For our health, we need to be able to receive support from our loved ones. Especially our woman friends. Friendships that nourish both parties in a reciprocal way that raise the vibration and fills each friend with gratitude and joy! These connections are a must! Men can be very supportive but often cannot engage with us in the same way as our female friends. They just can't! Many women get very frustrated with their men about this. But men's fiery sun-like nature has other purposes and gifts, like encouragement and motivation. If we need emotional support, these other fiery gifts naturally feel inappropriate in that moment. When we need feminine empathy and support, our man's fiery clarity or directional motivation or protection can feel like a mismatch. It often is! Here we find the feminine first and then we might connect up with our man a bit later having had the deeper support that we needed.

After connecting with Mother Earth and our inner self, it is our women friends who tend to be the best supporters. This of course is not always the case and it depends on the issue at hand too! But it tends to be our women friends or our bestie who will dance with us through life and hug us when life knocks us down and listen to us when we need to work stuff out and support us to try new things.

Support<u>er</u> or Support<u>ed</u> or Both?

Many women, due to the feminine wound, tend to give support out to others willingly but may find it difficult to receive it in return. Receiving support when we are at our most vulnerable... and our most feminine... can feel dangerous. How do you find receiving support? Do you receive it willingly? Or do you tend to get stuck in being a support for others?

Explore what beliefs you have about this. Is it safe for you to be vulnerable and humble? Or only for others to be vulnerable and humble? If this is the case, what do you fear happening if you let support in?

Receiving support can feel dangerous for some, as this is where we got hurt. This could be because there is a pattern of "not enough support", so when support does finally come into our life as an adult, we feel fear and resistance to it. We might be more identified with self-reliance. Notice what happens for you when others support you. Bring in self-compassion for your humanity and how you needed to survive.

Professional Support

As therapists and counsellors, it is unethical for us to have clients when we feel unsupported in our own lives. We have to commit to leading a supported life so that we can best support our clients. Part of this is being in Clinical Supervision. Supervisors are therapists with additional training, and their job is to support the therapist/client relationship. I believe this is the future of nursing, teaching and caring professions too, where needing support is currently seen as a weakness. These toxic systems are often, ironically, a danger to the people and children that these systems claim to serve. In reality, we all know that receiving support makes us stronger, healthier, more present and more loving.

Put Yourself First

Not in an egotistical way but in a sensible way that serves

the greater good. When we are fully supported both from within and by others, we are then in a position to help others. This is especially true of women. And even more so for mothers of young children. I go so far as to say that it is toxic for women to put others first. Yes, we might do this in an emergency but on a long-term basis it is incredibly unhealthy. Our own vessel must be filled in order for us to give. For men, with their naturally centrifugal and expansive energy, it is very different; a man will become energised by giving on a daily basis. He will feel more masculine, more energised and more potent. He will have to learn to rest, otherwise he will burn-out (such is the fire element). If he knows how to rest well – better still if he meditates too - he will do better by putting others first. But a woman? No way! She will feel exhausted at best and bitter at worst. For it is the job of the feminine to *receive* the wonders of life.

Some Support Tips

- I aim to be there *with* someone and not *for* someone.
- When I am supporting someone, I sense into my own body. As I'm with the other person, I notice my own feelings and sensations and how I am grounding. If I am standing, I notice if I need to sit down. If I am sitting, I sense into my sitting bones and my feet. Our own embodiment gives us support and gives space to others so that they automatically feel supported. When we do this we can also access our intuition more easily.
- Asking, "What do you need?" both to our self and to the other is incredibly useful and amazingly supportive.
- Allowing another's tears rather than rushing in with that hug to reassure the other can be very supportive. While well intended, invariably a hug interrupts their tears and

226

this could be a rare moment for them to let the tears flow. A few moments later we might want to offer them a hug. Conversely, another person may only be able to let go while they are being hugged. Usually this would be someone who is very close to us and who feels very safe with us. It's sometimes difficult to gauge. If in doubt, don't.

- What happens for you when you feel another's pain? Can you allow your own tears to flow while supporting others? To weep a little alongside them? This is true humanity. I'm not suggesting you fall apart and make it all about you, I'm suggesting you allow your tears to softly fall if they need to... to allow the fullness of the human moment to move through you at these times rather than to try and block your femininity in an ironic attempt to support another.

- Empathise by really sensing how the other might be feeling right now. If you can't get a sense, you might ask them, "Are you feeling disappointed/angry/sad?". Just this can feel very supportive. Even if our guess is wrong, it enables them to further clarify how they do actually feel.

- Depending on what type of support is needed, offer only what you can give. My best offerings are my therapeutic skills and the accompanying wisdom and knowledge, a good sandwich, a full English breakfast, a sleepover at my house, a Marie Kondo style declutter session, a walk in Nature. Another person's offering might be cooking or baking. Another might offer to do shopping or gardening or take the children somewhere for a few hours. I never offer support that I will resent giving and I never offer support that I haven't the resources to give. If we do this, it toxifies the gift as the other person has to then look after us on some level and this cancels out the deed. I once heard that to do this incurs a higher Karmic debt than to deliberately hurt someone!

- Give fully <u>and</u> know your limits. I have a friend who helps refugees. She is able to do this work as she knows when she's had enough and needs to stop. She spends a day resting in bed really blanketing herself and lets others cook for her. This is how she is able to do such challenging work - because she looks after herself. With her feminine power of support in balance, she finds she is able to remain feminine, nurturing and deeply compassionate.
- If you have kids, ask them what would support them in their life. Ask them if there is anything that they need that might make their life feel easier or more wonderful. They might suggest the latest tech or new shoes, and these may well be needed, but see if you can encourage them to sense deeper into their more emotional and practical needs. It might be more time with you or dad or an aunt or uncle... or more time in nature. Maybe they need more live music or would like to learn a simple instrument. My clients were not usually asked this kind of thing, so this is an insider's tip!
- It can really deepen our connection with our partner if we ask them what would support them in their life. "What can I do to support you this week with what you'd like to achieve?"

Support Prayer and Affirmation

You can adjust how you do this prayer and affirmation according to how much fire you need. (See Joy Prayer and Affirmation.) * Thank you for bestowing me with the wonderful power of support! * More and more I feel how Mother Earth supports me * I thankfully receive her energy and use it to further support myself! * Mother Earth under-stands me and constantly gives me energy * I connect with Earth's support more and more every day * I find many ways to support myself, and my powers of femininity blossom in my being! * I attract people into my life who support me and my feminine powers! * I allow others to support me more and more * As I am supported by Mother Earth and others, so I am able to support others more! * I embrace how feminine and supportive I am, just by breathing! * I support the workings of the universe by allowing my soul to shine through my feminine body and out into the world! *

I embrace how feminine and supportive I am, just by breathing! * I support the workings of the universe by allowing my soul to shine through my feminine body and out into the world!*...

...The boundaries of the feminine make life flow better. The earth element is the final densification of energy into form. It is the foundation; the solidity of form and structure; and as such, the earth element is all about boundaries and containment.

Chapter 12
Boundary

Boundary

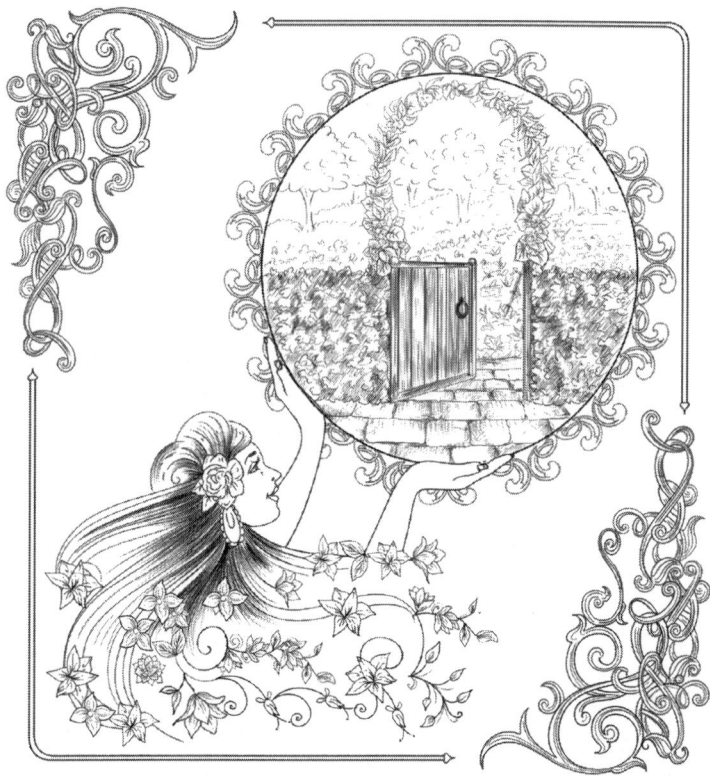

he boundaries of the feminine make life flow better. The earth element is the final densification of energy into form. It is the foundation; the solidity of form and structure; and as such, the earth element is all about boundaries and containment. The feminine is the keeper of boundary and form and, as such, women tend to be particularly good at holding things. Whether it's holding birthdates, regular family meal times, what goes in what recycling bin or making sure our friend who is unwell has a check-in call and so on. It is the boundary around her desires that shapes the world as we know it on a daily basis. The feminine power of boundary is what makes the world a better place.

Separate Yes, on One Level

We see the feminine power of boundary in Nature as the myriad structure and form that she takes. Every manifest "thing" has a boundary. There is an "edge" to it; where it begins and where it stops; whether it's the knobbly boundaries of a tree, the sharp and pointed edges of a blade of grass or the banks of the river. Unlike the water element, the earth element is a very dense energy that literally gives the *appearance* that everything is separate. It is so easy with the earth element energy to think that even we ourselves are separate from each other and everything else. And we *are* separate on one level and it's at this one level where it is incredibly important to get boundaries right, because when boundaries are foggy – on this one level – it can be a disaster.

And we are also *multi-dimensional* beings. We are not just physical beings. I believe that only a very small fraction of us is actually physical – that we are mostly energetic, and spiritual beings, physicalised into form in order to learn things and help this particular dimension evolve and develop.

233

She Rules the Physical

We feel this non-physical part of us most when our loved ones have the very same thoughts that we are having, or ring us when we think of them; and when we sense when someone is looking at us or if we might be in danger in a certain situation. But on a particular level we are indeed separate and we need this sense of separation to feel safe and healthy; and, indeed, so that others we interact with feel safe too. And this level is where the feminine rules!

On this human level of existence, when we get boundaries wrong, we know about it! A boundary breach is painful and confusing at best and terrifying at worst. Like a hole in an inkwell, poor boundaries can destroy a friendship or a family, ruin a business and can affect the health of everyone involved.

Different Levels of Boundaries

Sometimes boundaries are hard, like the structure that is our home and our front door and the bathtub that holds the bath water. Other boundaries are softer like the spider's web that denotes its home; and then there is the boundary that is the territory of a cat.

When it comes to ourselves there are many levels of boundary. We have our physical boundary that holds organs and systems, and even these have their own boundaries too. Then we have our emotional and intellectual boundaries. Further from this we have our psychic and a spiritual boundary.

Boundaries, Safety and Health

There are other sorts of boundaries that are important too – these are the contracts and agreements - whether spoken or unspoken.

We have relationship boundaries and business boundaries. All boundaries are vital to our sense of safety and security, and when boundaries are breached – crossed without permission, or not held in place with fiery clarity - this can have a serious effect.

Unclear or foggy boundaries cause all sorts of problems.

Boundaries for the Child

If an infant or child is given no clear boundaries then they don't feel safe and will either withdraw into their own world to find safety or will become extreme in their behaviour in an attempt to find a clear "edge". A baby will seek boundary and containment by searching for mother by reaching out with her electromagnetic field and with her eyes. If she doesn't get the attunement she needs, she will tend to remain in the etheric realms on one level until she can heal this as an adult. A toddler will run away from mother to experiment with separation but also so they can feel the comfort and delight of being held once again. Teenagers in particular unconsciously seek a boundary by trying out certain behaviours in order to test the strength of the container; "What will happen if I do this or if I do such and such?" Ideally, they discover that someone is in fact holding the boundary and under the commotion they end up feeling relief.

Bringing Up Kids

Creating daily boundaries helps make bringing up kiddies smooth and fun. I was a stay-at-home mum and the rhythm of the day saved me! But earning-money mums might find this helpful at weekends and holidays. Having set times for certain activities that always include tidying (to show that this is part of life) enables the day to run more smoothly. So for example breakfast might be at 7am and then play time and tidy-time for snack at 10am and then perhaps a walk afterwards and then lunch at 12.30 with washing up together and so on. This kind of thing contains a child (and a mum!) and helps them to feel secure and to feel safe with knowing – up to a point – how the day will flow. Maybe a sleep after lunch for both mum and child and then maybe visit a friend and then another tidy for snack at 4pm and so on until dinner and then bath time and bed. A rhythm like this means that there are less likely to be issues at bed time too. A candle at the table can make snack and meal times more peaceful with older children allowed to light or blow out the candle (taking care of course not to leave the candle unattended with or without the children). Certain activities can then be on certain days too. I did my washing on a Monday and we always visited a dear friend on a Tuesday with painting on a Thursday and so on. These further create boundary and containment and peace...

Older Kids...

Older children then have different boundaries of course with coming home from school or home-school activities and homework etc. Again, there is flexibility to all these rhythms and not a rigidity. They are containing and holding but not suppressing. All the time it helps if mum is checking what *she* needs. She can organise the day according to what supports *her* because if she is feeling supported and held then her kids will feel supported and held, and the whole world will then feel Right and Good and the boundaries will feel clear.

When Boundaries Fail

If boundaries are too tight we end up feeling controlled, suffocated and disempowered. Here the boundary has failed.

The autonomic nervous system will automatically want to take flight, fight, freeze or submit depending on how extreme the control is. These are the different involuntary reactions that we have no choice over until the system is healed. If a child receives over-rigid and fearful parenting she will no doubt tend to freeze or submit as an adult (and will need to find her "No" and her ability to stand her ground as an adult). Or the opposite pole might be true. Maybe we coped with rigid boundaries as a child by going into rebellion or domination of others in order to feel safe. Here, albeit ironically, we have equally lost touch with our empowerment, as when we live our whole life in a rebellious or controlling state, we are not truly free.

Exercise: Building a Physical Sense of Being Held – re-wiring the brain

- First and foremost, bring your self-compassion online. (Refresh how by reading the little paragraph in the Healing chapter about How to Heal Ourselves). Sense how this feels in your body.
- In a place of self-compassion so that your brain is wired for healing, find a blanket or shawl and wrap it round your shoulders – lengthwise (so the blanket or shawl is horizontal). Now, scrunching up the ends in each hand, fold your arms bringing your hands, complete with the shawl ends, under or near your marvellously warm armpits. So you are literally tucking yourself in.
- Then just sense inwards to how this feels. Sense into your pelvic bowl too to bring more support. And then just sense how it feels to be held... to feel the shawl round you – containing your shoulders and your arms and your hands. Notice how it feels to be held.

- You can also do this with your whole body – like a swaddle. It can feel like such a huge relief. It has to be experienced in order to really see how healing this exercise can be. Yes, we might look a bit daft but we have to heal ourselves and most of us have not been held in a way that was truly, deeply right for us. Now we are an adult and can listen to our deepest needs, we can swaddle our body to a level of perfection that our own mother could only have dreamed of achieving even if she did have that intention.
- You might want to experiment further with weighted blankets or, in tucking yourself into bed, place a few pillows on top of your quilt to add extra weight and a feeling of containment. Allow yourself and your inner child to really "clock" and register this feeling of "being held" and "boundary". Imagine the new connections firing up in your brain; the new "being held" wiring replacing the old outdated "un-held" wiring of your childhood. Breathe deeply into your belly, feeling your lower belly expand when you inhale and shrink as you let all the old air out.
- Do this as often as is necessary until you don't need it any more.

Healing Boundary Issues

Working with self-compassion is the first step to healing the deep feelings of lostness, sadness and fear that come with a boundary-less childhood; when we didn't feel held or weren't held *enough* by our mother in loving presence. I show people who have had little holding or containment as children how to "self-swaddle" with a lovely blanket to build the experience of being properly held and contained in a loving way. If we weren't held enough as a child it will naturally feel awkward to hold ourselves or our inner child as an adult as it goes against the grain. It doesn't feel natural. (The super ego will also tend to humiliate or shame us in an attempt to keep us the same.) We can experiment and learn to re-wire ourselves. We can talk to our super ego and reassure it that it is safe to change, and we can talk to our inner child acknowledging how difficult it was back then and how we survived it all. In doing this, we are showing our little inner child true *interconnectedness* which feels even *better* than anything our mother could have done, as no one knows better than ourselves what we really, deeply need.

Escaping Old Rigidity

To heal the wounds of too rigid parenting we might want to work with setting up little "escaping" scenarios thus reminding our nervous system how free it can be these days – as opposed to when we were a defenceless child and dependent on our parents. Escaping from the sofa to the kitchen to make a cup of tea, or escaping the kitchen to the bathroom to go to the loo, or escaping the house to go to the shop to buy a loaf of bread. These "nano escapes" can utilise the flight system and can feel very empowering. When I go to the dentist, I always park a good 500 yards away and then, once the treatment is finished, I "escape" to my car. I literally run away. This literally "runs off" the stress hormones that were released into my bloodstream during the dental treatment where I had to override my natural inclination to escape. This not only feels very freeing afterwards, but I also find it avoids that feeling of disconnectedness or "depression" that happens throughout the rest of the day if I don't do this (this is the impact of the stress hormones being left in the system as they haven't been run off). This is helpful to do after any invasive treatment or procedure that we felt we had to "endure".

NB If these types of escapes feel too activating, then you might want to work with a trauma-aware therapist or counsellor who can work with you more slowly.

Expressing Needs and Preferences Leads to Clearer Boundaries

Which duty and responsibility belongs to whom? Muddled and foggy boundaries cause so many problems! Problems at home and the workplace and within relationships are always due to foggy boundaries of some sort. Here, a deeper exploration using the feminine power of relationship to discover the deeper human needs is what can help. "What do I *really* need right now?" is a fine question to ask ourselves in any moment and can help to clarify things, as is asking the other person what they *really* need. Maybe they need to feel seen in some way that hasn't happened yet? Or to be appreciated? Here a boundary confusion can instantly clarify. If we are the ones that have stepped over a line, what did we really need, deep down, that caused us to do that? Or conversely, if it's someone else "stepping on our toes" because of their own boundary fudge, then what did they really need in doing that? When we relate with each other this way, with curiosity and openness and compassion for the human condition, the boundary simply *becomes* clear and doesn't have to be artificially constructed in some way.

Boundary Violation

Boundary violations often happen with force, but this force is not always physical. Either way there is a "breach" of some kind – an invasion; someone steals our handbag, or burgles our home, or we are attacked or shouted at. These are all violations, as force is being used in some way against us. As I was writing this, someone posted on my local neighbourhood WhatsApp group how a man tried to tempt a 12-year-old girl to get into his van. Her autonomic nervous system kicked in with her going into full "flight" as she ran to her grandmother's house to safety.

240

Here, she found her "no" and her healthy nervous system worked quickly and efficiently to get her to a safe place. If she was greeted welcomingly and without blame, this girl will not be traumatised from this event, but might even feel empowered as a result of her ability to escape unharmed. Sometimes, if we have experienced a lot of trauma (where we could not escape a violation as we were too young or too vulnerable or where we were not supported properly afterwards) our autonomic nervous system may automatically freeze in situations that remind us of these early events in some way. Healing our nervous system by finding our "no" and by enabling the flight and fight system is a sure way to get our sense of empowerment and sense of boundary back again.

The Masculine Protects the Boundary

Whilst the feminine is the boundary itself, the *protector* of the boundary is the fiery masculine. It is the fiery dynamism of the masculine that is the *enforcer* of that boundary and the protector of the receptive vulnerability. The fire element does this with his fiery clarity, expression of needs or with dynamic action. All the boundaries in the world can be beautifully in place but if they are not *protected* and *upheld* with our fiery speech and clarity then we have problems.

The Inner and Outer Protector

In a co-dependent situation a woman may leave her man to do all the protecting but this is not healthy. Yes, men, being so fiery and like the Sun, do tend to be quick to protect. This is both natural and noble and vital for the polarity and chemistry of the polarity relationship. But in health, a woman must know how to be empowered herself **as well** so that she can feel safe within herself and not *have* to depend on her man (or in a same-sex relationship, depend on the more fiery woman). It's about being whole and having choices. In health, we are able to stand our ground and get behind our speech and dynamic action and yet also be able to surrender into our feminine and feel safe and protected by the additional presence of our man. But it's a fine balance in the polarity relationship! If a man isn't protective enough – the woman will have to "man-up" and the polarity will flatten to a boring drone...

Sensing the edge...

In a friendship or workplace situation, where a breach might be more subtle, we might say, "Ooh, hang on a minute, something feels 'off' here." Or, "I think this is outside of our agreement." Both these examples are still the fire element working healthily and expressing easily. This is why it is so vital that little girls are allowed to find their "no" – this is their inner masculine developing which will help them to protect their own boundaries as a child and as a woman out in the world (this in turn also helps us to truly find our "yes!").

The Solar Plexus Warns Us

On a subtle level, we tend to get a twinge in the fiery stomach/ solar plexus when something is "off" - when a boundary is being crossed. This is our fire element "sparking" in our body and showing us that we need to protect a boundary by speaking up. We might even hold our hand up in front of our solar plexus to denote that a boundary needs holding in place. If we have not been supported as children to protect our boundaries and had our boundaries violated, our solar plexus might have shut down or might feel numb. When this happens, we are not able to sense that warning twinge within us and might find that we keep getting into situations regarding boundary violations. With our own development we can reconnect to our "no' and to our power and awaken our threat brain to work properly, allowing this innate protective system – which includes the solar plexus – to come back online.

Her Standards are Higher

There is an irony here as it is the masculine that is the protector of boundaries yet it is also the masculine that is more likely to cross a boundary. Men, having incarnated as a representative of the masculine principle, are naturally protective; but also, in being like the Sun, can be indiscriminate in their fieriness. We see this in the Sun with its constant reactivity and how it throws out its solar flares with no sense of the consequences. But this is the nature of fire. Complaining about this is like complaining that fire is hot or that water is wet. And... it is usually women who draw the line with bad behaviour. The masculine – left unchecked – is a particularly powerful and dynamic energy that simply *is* more likely to leap out and cross a boundary. Men do better in life with a woman to keep them in check or with a partner with higher standards and women do better in life when they allow men to develop. But it's a fine balance. If her standards are too high she might exhaust her man! It's a delicate balance and all about development...

He Polishes up to Her Standard...

The feminine has always been "the line in the sand" for the masculine. She is the one who shapes life as we know it. The masculine, in wanting to naturally serve the feminine, will tend to "polish up" to please the feminine and will willingly fall in line to impress her. We see this with the male peacock, who has to go to a lot of trouble in order to impress the pea-hen! And sometimes she is still not impressed. He has to try harder and look how amazing he becomes. Tales of the Wild West describe what it was like when it was just men there and no women; where the behaviour of the men was likened to that of wild animals. But as soon as the women started showing up, things began to change. The men started scrubbing up and combing down their hair and changing their behaviour. They knew that they had to behave around the women if they wanted any female attention! In this world, the feminine holds the boundaries around sex, behaviour and pretty much everything else!

Low Standards?

If a woman has low standards then this can be a disaster for society as he can't then polish *up*. If she accepts bad behaviour, then there is no development. Development comes as she sets her standards high by declaring her needs and desires and enabling him to then clearly see what is expected of him. He then gets the chance to polish up and become "a better man". And men love this! Men are not like women at all! Women so often can't be bothered with a challenge as we have too much to do but men get to feel themselves as a man when they have a challenge. This is how men develop and grow. With a woman with high standards, they have to strategise and think and use their determination to impress her and in doing this they get to feel amazing. When a woman sets her standards high, everyone wins and society gets to develop.

Learning to Walk Off

If he is behaving badly – which men are prone to do, as fire is like that – you can walk away for an hour or so or even for longer (whatever it takes). Although dramatic, it powerfully gives him the space to re-think and improve. Men often need some sort of "jeopardy" in order to grow and our walking off and giving him space provides this jeopardy. If he is worth his salt, he will realise what he has done and will quickly want to make amends. He will thank you, as this helps him develop and he knows it. The space created by you gives him the time to think about his behaviour and the causes of it and gives you the space to work on your own healing. If he is a good match for you he will love you even more, and the new boundary clarification will come out of the ensuing conversation. If he is not a good match for you, you can both move on, and thereupon a new boundary is agreed and you are then free to find a man who is more willing to develop and grow and who will adore you with your higher standards and your amazing feminine energy! Holding our standards high and being willing to walk off when he is behaving badly does take fire. It's masculine principle stuff; walking away and feeling your own empowerment as you hold and insist upon the amazing feminine standard.

Other Relationship Boundaries

Every relationship has various agreements that function as boundaries within that relationship – they define the type of relationship that it is. These agreements, although often unconscious, enable us to feel safe within that relationship. We know where we stand. Certain behaviours are expected and allowed, and within certain types of relationships, when a boundary is crossed, we might feel rage, anger and a sense of betrayal with the deeper feelings hiding underneath of fear, confusion and disappointment. All relationships and groups feel safer in that dynamic when the boundaries are named. "You are my new friend!" we might say. Or, "I love having you as my husband/wife/lover!" Or, "I so appreciate our colleagueship." I know some people who have friends that they travel with, others that they read poetry with and others that they make love with. As long as the boundaries are agreed it feels peaceful in our hearts.

Boundaries are Negotiable.

If a boundary is not negotiable then it is a failed boundary. Boundaries by their nature help us to feel safe and secure so if we feel unsafe then this is a sign that the boundary is too tight or too loose and someone will be feeling unseen and unheard in some way. Adjusting boundaries can feel rather delicate as it touches on our own personal violations or betrayals that we might have experienced in the past or as a child. Skilled negotiation and compassion are needed for everyone concerned to feel seen and heard and therefore trusted, and for the true boundary to organically appear out of the confusion.

Women and Men Fudge Boundaries Differently

Women and men tend to mess up boundaries in different ways. Men being so fiery and like the Sun can be more "reactive" and can make rash moves or decisions like solar flares. In its worst negative expression this might be followed up by intellectual justifications and rationalisations for taking such actions. Women being like Nature might cross a boundary in a much more subtle or hidden way. We tend to be more like ivy or like water seeping through a tiny hole so we might subtly take over or unconsciously use our nurturing power to interfere (I trip on this one frequently!). We might gossip and breach a boundary, or have lots of dark thoughts about someone (which is a psychic boundary violation), or we may attempt to lure a man from his wife – breaching a marital boundary. The feminine in general tends to be less direct. But when the feminine power of boundary is used well, there is *relationship* and *relating* which naturally includes *hearing* what the

246

human needs are of the people involved. The feminine power of
Relationship naturally resolves boundary disputes on any level. No
one gets hurt when the feminine power of boundary is used well.

On Becoming Exhausted

Women, due to their innate power of nurturing and support, can find
it difficult to hold certain boundaries regarding their own needs. We
might keep caring and caring until exhaustion and bitterness set in.
Also "hardness" – where her inner masculine has had to "muscle up" to
protect tender emotions and feelings that are not allowed expression.
This suppression of the feminine is deeply embedded in our culture
and in the systems that have been created to "take care of us"; where
the masculine "just do it" and "power-on" is encouraged in women,
and her core tenderness and emotionality is seen as an inconvenience,
at best. Here a woman can feel dead inside and as if she is betraying
herself. The most important boundary a woman has is the one
surrounding her own personal needs! Due to its receptive and
gravitational energy, the feminine has to learn to protect herself by
knowing her own boundaries and her own limits. She has to learn
to get super clear about what she needs and what she desires. Being
as nurturing and caring as she is can mean that she puts herself last
on the list and this is quite toxic for a woman.

Putting Ourselves First

The feminine is foundational. It is the fertile ground out of
which everything is born. When the feminine is "in place"
everything then flows from this and life is good for everyone.
I'm going to say that again: **When the feminine is "in place"
everything then flows from this and life is good for everyone.**
*The feminine is foundational. It is the fertile ground out of which
everything is born.*

Life is good for everyone when the feminine is joyful, well loved-up and happy. Our whole life changes when we begin to put ourselves first. This is counter to what we have been taught. This is because the masculine is the opposite! The masculine gets energy from *giving*! We have been brought up with half of this natural law missing: that women must receive and take care of themselves in order to keep charged and healthy. I'm not talking about narcissism here; I'm not talking about that selfish need to be always the centre of attention and "me, me, me" all the time. I'm talking about our innate and natural magnetic energy that gets really affected if it's not energised by self-care or being given to. It's our feminine responsibility to check that we are filled up before we care; nourished before we nurture; and generally having a joy-filled and empleasured life before we consider sharing our energy. We need to use the feminine power of boundary to keep our joy and pleasure levels high.

Exercise: Saying No
- Sit in a chair and sense into your feet on the floor and sense into your sitting bones. This anchors and grounds you.
- When you feel grounded and anchored, see how it feels to raise your hands in front of you, with your palms facing outwards away from you. Imagine there is something in front of you that you really don't want. (Try not to imagine something too challenging here – keep it simple, like a plate of food that you don't like.)
- Here, you are holding a boundary. Sense the gap between the back of your hands and the front of your body.
- Feel how it feels to hold your hands up like this in front of you. Feel how it feels to maintain it. (Keep grounding by sensing your feet and sitting bones or sense into your pelvic basin for more support) You can experiment here with

- moving your hands even further away from you – using even more power – and then notice how it is to bring your hands back towards you.
- Try saying out loud "No," or, "No thanks."
- Keep noticing what is happening in your body as you do this. Don't speed up. Keep it slow. If something feels overwhelming then consider finding a therapist or counsellor who can help you work through this.
- If you do practice this, how does it feel to do this? Sense into your body for any heat... Heat, flushing or "burning" is great as it's your fire igniting within you. Notice what your breathing does too; fire needs air. If you start yawning a lot, this is great as its your inner "bellows" getting going! Allow yawning fully as this also releases the jaw and tension in the skull which is how we might block our fire to our head and eyes. Yawning is the release and reorganisation of the energies and the five elements so allow it freely!
- If you don't feel anything this is still important as it shows you that you may well need to practice this a lot in order to awaken your fire. Be curious. Observe what you discover about yourself.

The Super Ego Stops Us Saying No

While I was editing this chapter, my dear friend Rebecca called. She wondered if I would like to walk with her. I so wanted to connect with her! I hadn't seen her for what felt like an age and yet I wanted to finish this chapter. Writing this chapter was challenging enough without having this additional dilemma! Well, you can see I would be tempted! But I could feel I would be betraying myself if I did. But I just couldn't seem to find my, "I'd love to but I need to finish this chapter on boundaries first." I found myself offering a good chat instead (which was still not what I really desired). After a while she realised that she needed a walk even more than she needed a chat with me, so we agreed to meet the next day.

Super Ego Causes Guilt and Shame

She had saved me here but I felt guilty. Knowing guilt is one of the calling cards of the super ego; I knew I had been under super ego attack (See this information in the "Feminine Power of Joy" chapter). Here I could then remember what it had been saying: "Oh I haven't seen her for ages!" "I am neglecting her," and the crux: "She won't be your friend anymore!" The feeling of guilt coincided with a tension in my solar plexus. So I said to my super ego – mine always appears to be on my right, "Hey, it's okay, I know you are scared about Rebecca but I've got this, we will see her tomorrow and have much more fun." Here my super ego was silenced and suitably reassured and then I got right back on my computer to write this.

Not Betraying Myself...

My super ego was attempting to break a boundary I had made with myself (to finish my book) to protect me from Rebecca "dumping me", and yet I knew that Rebecca's and my friendship was way deeper than that and that she would not want me to betray myself. Here though, was a vital point I had missed out of the chapter, and Rebecca's phone call was incredibly timely. Thanks to her I was reminded how the super ego might – through fear – cause us to abandon our self and drop a boundary. Here we might end up over-nurturing/caring for others to the neglect of our own needs, thus breaking an internal agreement and then feeling really rotten. Or, indeed in another situation, the super ego could persuade us to cross a boundary and then justify it.

Better Boundaries than our Mother

If as a child, we were not shown how to hold our own boundary, then certain boundaries may feel weak or even unknown to us. Or the opposite pole could be true where our boundaries may be "rigid" and our behaviour controlling as an overcompensation. This makes sense when we understand that the feminine power of boundaries contains, holds and thus nurtures us in our daily life and within all of our relationships. So, it makes further sense that we "rigidify" and control in an attempt to feel held and supported. We can see here how we need to be compassionate with ourselves and with others if there is rigidity or controlling behaviour.

Controlling and Rigid are Boundary Failures

When we find ourselves becoming controlling and rigid, this is when a boundary is failing. Boundaries are *always* negotiable. Controlling and rigid is when there is old fear in our body. Here we can pause and take a breath. Where is the fear in the body? Can we express our fear to the other person? We can bring in more support by sensing our sitting bones and the pelvic basin. From this place of self-connection and support, we may find it easier to come back into relationship with the other by expressing our vulnerability, hearing their response and then, with communication and hearing, we might be able to find the natural boundary.

Sometimes it's only through being in a therapeutic relationship that we can heal the early traumas that left us so un-boundaried or rigid.

Deep Diving for Our Human Needs

Meanwhile, it is important to practice deep-diving for our needs and our preferences. If we were brought up feeling unsupported this will take a lot of practice and oodles of self-compassion (we can only heal when we are in a state of self-compassion). Once we are in a state of self-compassion we can ask, "What do I need right now?" or we can ask the other person, "What do you need right now?" This is the birth of boundary.

Some Boundary Tips

- When two people discover and verbalise their deepest needs to each other the healthy boundary naturally appears.
- If you find that you tend to cross boundaries by dealing with things that are not yours to deal with or by responding to things that are not yours to respond to, ask yourself two things: what do I really need? Who showed me this behaviour in my childhood? Remember self-compassion...
- When you are in conflict with another, you can use the feminine power of boundary to clarify what the deep human needs are that caused the boundary issue. Deep down, somebody needs something here that is not being expressed.
- Get used to acknowledging the subtle twinge in the solar plexus area that alerts us of a boundary cross.
- Be willing to lovingly turn down a friend or loved one. They will trust you more as they will know that when you say "yes", you mean it, so they will be able to relax with you more. When I say no to something, right after, I always try and find something else that we can both say yes to.
- If you are amongst friends, and conversation slides into gossiping, then, without judgement, see if you can change the subject. Your pals will notice and will trust you more,
- When you are invited to do something, practice saying, "Ooo... let me just check how that feels..." In the space you've created, you can check your needs and you will be showing your pal how to do the same in future.

- If you find yourself in a conversation or a situation that makes your solar plexus twinge, have a go at saying, "I notice I'm feeling uncomfortable."
- Slowing things down is always useful with boundary checking; whether it's during designing a garden, during lovemaking or arranging a holiday. If one person feels uncomfortable, then slowing things down gives everyone the chance to connect with themselves and see what they need. It's about creating safety for everyone. "Let's pause a minute" is a useful thing to say. If you feel uncomfortable about something, the chances are the other person does too.

The clearer we are with our boundaries, the healthier we are and the more influential we become.

Boundary Prayer and Affirmation

You can adjust how you do this prayer and affirmation according to how much fire you need. (See Joy Prayer and Affirmation.)* As a woman I begin to enjoy clarifying boundaries! * Life becomes easier as I attend to this * I find clear boundaries everywhere I go! * If I cross a boundary I feel able to make amends and check what my actual needs are * I am more able to see when I am crossing a boundary and I am compassionate with myself when I do this * And I am more able to see when others might cross a boundary * When others cross a line and I am affected I am more able to see when compassion is needed and when I need to stand my ground and say "no." * My solar plexus talks to me and shows me when a boundary needs clarifying *

So, the nub ...

It amazes me; how in spite of masked and persistent agendas, the fabric of society is still woven according to feminine influences and desires, whether we are consciously aware of this or not. Yes, certain forces have sought for millennia to undermine this – with so many systems and organisations set up to disempower us and steer all humans away from our true power. But, within the family, and in the community; in everyday life, the feminine in both women and men has still managed to influence left, right and centre. We see the microcosm of this so clearly with how a woman will arrange her home; even if she chooses to have it "unarranged" it is still usually her choice, and her man will tend to follow suit (or rebel against it if she is too controlling). The feminine is busy shaping culture by desiring and choosing a new way of doing things; home births, organic food, eating less meat, recycling, plastic-free and local shopping, home and alternative education, and healing using nature's bounty together with the intelligence of the human energy field.

It is here that - as incarnations of the feminine, as huge influencers of our world - we must take time to check what it is we desire, and know this deeply in our hearts. If we fall into "demanding" we become the negative aspect of the feminine – controlling and rigid. The goddess is never controlling or rigid and it would serve the whole world well if we were to become more embodied in the many ways of the feminine. But to do this with full success, we must know our masculine; we must know our fire, our clarity and our empowered self. This way, we are adults, fully influential and potentialized women living as nature and God intended. The men then, can return to their original purpose – that of being more like The Knight; serving the feminine and giving to the feminine in order to delight her;

and in so doing bring about his fuller sense of meaning and purpose. Peace is so possible on this Earth.

Times are challenging indeed. For millennia, polarity has been used to manipulate the populace – to turn us all against each other – men and women against each other and against themselves. This has created incredible suffering and immeasurable misery. How can I myself help? All I can do is show people how we can use polarity to heal our bodies and our hearts, our relationships and our communities.

All human beings have incredible potential. We don't tend to know this, it's the nature of the beast that we have to actually *be* at a new level of consciousness in order to know its nature. And, unlike a business plan or our garden design, we can't tell how the next step will feel or what it will be like. We can *imagine* it but we don't know until we are there.

Humans tend to think we are fairly well developed as we are. I remember someone saying that, "... we are perfect just as we are, yes, but we are not complete." We are unfinished; if we were truly complete, we would perhaps be in a state of constant joy, sublime spiritual ecstasy, and maybe even not need to incarnate.

Part of this "unfinished" is that we are still not fully aware of our multi-dimensionality. This level that we exist in is not really separate from all the other levels and even from the Source itself. It appears separate due to the feminine power of boundary, but we have all of the other frequencies within us and it is these frequencies that we can experience when we meditate or when we are in certain states of mind.

Another aspect of this "unfinished" is that trauma - old energy that hasn't yet been able to integrate and be discarded - lowers our vibration and keeps us in survival mode, preventing us from reaching the higher states of consciousness that we are capable of.

But for many years now, people have been healing their trauma and this is having the effect of raising not only the individual's vibration but also that of the whole collective too. What enables this process is allowing ourselves to feel through the old pain we are carrying and thus transform it. At the same time, we have never been so medicated; but in spite of this mass attempt to anaesthetise our pain with drugs, many of us are stepping forward to heal ourselves anyway. Women are being called on to be very different from their grandmothers. Men are being equally invited to stand up and do things very differently from their grandfathers.

Women embodying into their feminine body is a vital step. It's foundational to the development of humanity. As women, we *are* the foundation; earth and water. We are the bricks, the glue; the mud. The process starts here – at the base. In the physical body we see this reflected in the chakra system; with the first and second chakras (earth and water) energy centres being at our own base; our perineum (earth chakra) and just above the clitoris (water chakra). The next chakra up is fire - the masculine – in the belly. From here the energy jumps up a level to the air chakra – in the heart, to the ether chakra in the throat and then up to the brow and crown chakras.

The more we embody into our femininity and surrender and *enjoy* our feminine energy, the more we enable the next level of shift ... and the next stage can unfurl ...

Divine Polarity

I see our future with more polarity. Not polarity as in duality and polarisation, but Divine Polarity. In my field of work, it is very noticeable that the more women heal their trauma the more feminine they become. And the more men heal their trauma the more masculine they become. Simultaneous to this is the igniting of the inner opposite force; so women tend to become more empowered right alongside their blossoming femininity, and men become more receptive and open as they become more magnificently masculine. Through this continual healing of trauma coupled with the realising of our true human capacity that comes with this great awakening that we are all part of, I see health for all of us will be a normal state of being. The levels of electricity caused by the polarity will raise couples up to incredible heights of ecstasy. I see new higher levels of relationship, love and spiritual attainment with the Divine Neutral Principle coming into being; where polarity returns to God – the Source, and All That Is.

And I leave it here, saying how I hope you have enjoyed reading about and experimenting with your feminine powers. I wish you well on your journey of discovering the fullness of your femininity and indeed your power to protect it.

With an open and God-filled heart,
Catherine

With Thanks

To my parents for being radical. To my beautiful and wise big sister, Mandy, who reads everything and for suggesting I "hurry up and get on with it!". To my teachers, especially Dianne Vanness. To Clare Kavanagh for your incredible vision and for "seeing" me. To Anna Walker for The Bowl. To Rebecca – my Japanese partner in crime who has been totally there with me especially during these past three years. To my friend Liz whose love of polarity is so inspiring and for her incredible expertise on boundaries and for reading the whole manuscript *twice*! To Neil Lawson, for his Vision Board workshop, keen observation and for reading the second manuscript and seeing its importance to the world. To my beautiful friend Amy for reading the early version whilst on holiday in France and for her amazing Virgoan eye regarding the illustrations and the beauty and ease of the final design. To the amazing Ana Gracey for your long-term deep and wonderful friendship throughout which has included incredible tech support and marvellous editing and for suggesting that Vicky look through an early version of the manuscript. Thank you, Vicky, for your thought-provoking questions and for your engagement with the book – you were incredibly helpful! To Bill and Rowan for your endless years of patience and for believing in me and giving me the space to write. Next to hugely appreciate is Dawn Larder on People Per Hour - the Spanish Queen whose illustrations make the book incredibly special – you were so patient and such fun to work with as we experimented with so many ways of illustrating pleasure in particular! To Sue Parlby, for additional help with the illustrations. And then Keith, my marvellous expat editor again from People Per Hour as well as Cyprus, Arizona and the Seven Seas too it seems! Thank you for your incredible patience, understanding and great communication style. It has been fun!

And to my dear friend and neighbour Diane, for letting the Divine speak through you and for many evening ponderings on illustrations and cover-design queries. And "Bazzie" of In The Dog House Design, the heaven-sent book designer and twin sister of the Spanish Queen illustrator (what a team you make!) who so efficiently and smoothly made this book "breathe" and flow so smoothly and feel wonderful to read. And to my dear clients, past and present. You have taught me so much and I feel such gratitude to have met you and worked with you. I love you all. And lastly to Tony; to have met you has changed my life. Your grounded, Taurean observance of what needs to be done, coupled with your steadfast and determined fire has totally enabled the completion of this project.

Additional thanks and appreciation go to the authors and teachers who have more recently inspired me to write about this information and they are Laura Doyle and her work in "ending world divorce", Mark Gungor and his work that includes *Laugh Your Way to a Better Marriage: a Tale of 2 Brains* and Tony Robbins. All have been very courageous and I am indebted to them.

Printed in Great Britain
by Amazon